MW00875036

NEXT LEVEL COOKBOOK

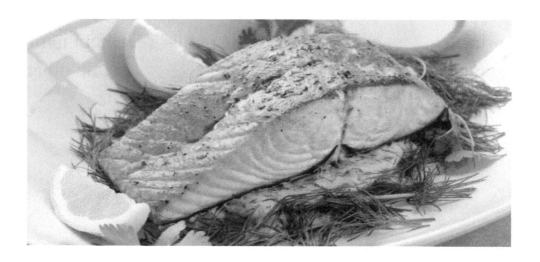

Over 40+ Delicious Recipes for Optimal Health During Menopause Inspired by Stacy T. Sims and Selene Yeager's Teachings

Jacqueline Parish

Copyright©2024 by Jacqueline Parish

All rights reserved. No part of this publication may be reproduced, distributed or transmitted in any form, or by any means, including photocopying, recording, or other electronic or mechanical methods, without prior written permission from the publisher, except in the case of brief quotations embodied in critical reviews and certain other non-commercial uses permitted by copyright law.

Disclaimer

The information in this book is intended for educational purposes only and is not a substitute for professional medical advice. Always consult with your physician before making any changes to your diet especially if you have any underlying health conditions.

The recipes in this book are based on Stacy T. Sims and Selene Yeager's teachings but are not directly endorsed by her. While this recipe is designed to promote optimal health and hormone balance, results may vary.

INTRODUCTION

Welcome to the heart and soul of the kitchen, where each dish not only nourishes the body but also the spirit, and every recipe tells a story. I welcome you to join me in enjoying the beauty of food and its ability to assist us through life's transformations as we set off on this culinary adventure together.

This cookbook is a tribute to the bravery and tenacity of women navigating the uncharted waters of menopause, not merely a compilation of dishes. It's a cozy hug and a gentle reminder that you're not travelling alone and that, even in the middle of your hormonal ups and downs, the kitchen can be your safe refuge and shelter.

Stacy T. Sims and Selene Yeager knowledge inspires the preparation of a variety of hearty recipes in these pages.

We have carefully created every cuisine, from filling stews to colorful salads, rich desserts to substantial soups, to nourish both your body and spirit throughout this metamorphic period.

This cookbook aims to nourish not just your body but also your soul, savoring the simple pleasures of a home-cooked meal with loved ones, and discovering joy in the kitchen. It's about finding beauty in the middle of change and accepting the changes that come with going through menopause with thankfulness and grace.

So, my dear friends, I want you to welcome the voyage with an open heart and an adventurous spirit as you turn the pages and set out on your own culinary experiences. I hope these recipes uplift, soothe, and nurture your spirit from the inside out.

UNDERSTANDING MENOPAUSE

The term menopause entered the English language in 1821, credited to French physician Charles-Pierre-Louis de Gardanne. Combining the words meno, which means "month" and has to do with the moon, and pause, which means to stop anything, the phrase literally indicates the conclusion of your monthly cycle.

Menopause was a major source of uncertainty long before the term was defined. Early Greek and Roman doctors believed that if a woman did not discharge the toxins and poisons from her body during menopause, which ended with the monthly loss of blood due to menstruation, she would go insane.

Treatments for this supposed "menopausal madness" have ranged throughout time from bizarre to barbaric, involving anything from imprisoning women in asylums to extracting toxins with leeches. For a very long time, menopausal treatments were very different and ineffective because nobody knew what was actually happening in the body (ovarian failure) to create symptoms and, most of the time, accelerate the end of a woman's cycle.

Researchers didn't start focusing on the endocrine system, particularly the ovaries, and the presence of hormones as the keys to comprehending the causes of menopause until the late 1800s and early 1900s. During this same period, researchers introduced the first oral remedies to address menopausal symptoms. These treatments were simple formulations made from processed animal ovarian tissue. Some of these treatments appeared to improve hot flashes, what was then called "sexual dysfunction" (current medicine refers to it as hypoactive sexual desire disorder, or low libido), or painful sex, both commonly encountered in menopause.

American chemists Edgar Allen and Edward Doisy were the first to isolate the main hormone generated by the ovaries in 1923. Doisy would go on to receive the Nobel Prize for his discovery of the chemical makeup of vitamin K.

Research demonstrated that this hormone, also known as primary ovarian hormone, stimulates reproductive system functions linked to a woman's menstrual cycle. A few years later, we would all familiarly refer to it as estrogen. The phrase originates from the terms estrus and gen, symbolizing the formation of a monthly cycle. I'm just dropping in to let you know that, yes, it would be easy to brush all of these aside as pointless historical minutiae.

However, these findings essentially laid the groundwork for our current understanding of how estrogen influences menstruation and pregnancy, as well as how its relative lack of estrogen triggers menopause.

By 1933, they were producing and prescribing estrogen under the brand name Emmenin. It was made initially from placenta extracts and then from pregnant women's urine. It was used to treat menopausal symptoms and dysmenorrhea, or pain throughout the menstrual cycle. It was eventually modified using pregnant mares' urine and given the brand Premarin, which the FDA first approved for sale in 1942. With Premarin's entry into the hormone therapy market, a decades-long debate about the efficacy of hormone-based treatments for menopausal symptoms and associated disorders would begin.

PRESENT DAY

Menopause, which signifies the end of a woman's ability to procreate as well as the end of her monthly periods, is an important biological milestone in her life. It usually happens between the ages of 45 and 55, with 51 being the average age.

During this phase, the ovaries progressively decrease the amount of estrogen and progesterone they produce, which are essential hormones that govern the menstrual cycle and enhance fertility. This hormonal decline brings on menopausal symptoms, a set of physical and psychological changes that vary greatly in severity and duration among women.

The first stage of the menopausal process is the perimenopause, a transitional period characterized by irregular menstrual cycles and symptoms like hot flashes, night sweats, mood swings, and altered sleep habits. Women gradually achieve menopause, which is defined as the lack of menstruation for 12 consecutive months, as their menstrual cycles grow more irregular.

After menopause, women enter the postmenopausal stage, which includes the years after the last menstrual cycle.

A wide range of feelings and views influenced by societal attitudes, individual beliefs, and personal experiences commonly accompany the menopause, which is not simply a biological process but also a significant psychosocial and cultural phenomenon. Menopause signifies the conclusion of a woman's reproductive cycle and a new chapter in her life, presenting opportunities for personal growth, self-exploration, and rejuvenation.

Menopause, which signifies the end of a woman's reproductive journey and the beginning of a new chapter marked by wisdom, resilience, and the possibility of sustained personal and professional fulfillment, is ultimately a normal and inevitable aspect of the aging process for women.

THE CHANGE

Menopause, as defined medically, is the year that passes after your last menstrual period. In other words, you must wait a full year after your last menstrual period to consider your final period truly final, as confirmation is only possible if you have missed your period for a year or longer. You will then officially be considered postmenopausal.

Although this seems logical from a clinical standpoint, in real life, this paradigm can be very perplexing, and with good reason. People often describe menopause as a one-time event that starts on a specific day, much like menstruation did a few decades ago. You might assume that your menstrual cycle will end abruptly one day.

Many women who have experienced menopause may grin wryly at this, knowing better. Menopause is actually a dynamic, sometimes protracted process that may last for many years rather than a single day. Additionally, whatever your prior definition of normalcy may have been, it is currently in a state of flux and change throughout this time.

Menopause Development: Ages and Stages:

Medical textbooks have only recently begun to define the intricacy of the menopausal transition; some now characterize menopause as occurring in numerous phases. To put it more briefly, we are investigating pre-menopause, perimenopause, and post-menopause.

Pre-menopause:

For as long as your menstrual cycle is regular, you are in the premenopausal or "reproductive" stage. Puberty marks the beginning of it, and the menopause marks its conclusion.

Perimenopause

You are approaching the menopause transition, also known as the perimenopause, after your menstruation starts to become irregular. Your menstruation may act a little strange at first. It could manifest as something heavier or lighter, appear earlier or later, last longer or shorter, or become more or less unpleasant. Put differently, there won't be consistency because everything is up for grabs.

After a while, it won't appear at all for at least two months. Hot flushes, changes in mood, cognition, and sleep quality are all more likely to occur during this period, and even the most courageous among us could feel like they've spent too much time at the fair. Forty-seven is the average age at which perimenopause begins, however this might vary based on lifestyle variables, genetics, and ethnicity. Though it might take up to fourteen years, the transformation typically lasts four to eight years.

Post menopause:

You are deemed postmenopausal if it has been a complete year since your last menstrual cycle. But let's imagine that after a year without a period, all of a sudden you get one, the clock resets, and you find yourself back in perimenopause! You'll start over and build your way back up to the postmenopausal stage.

Crucially, although this isn't always the case, symptoms usually begin to lessen or stop a few years following the last menstrual cycle.

Menopause often strikes women between the ages of forty and fifty-eight, with the average age at menopause being between fifty-one and fifty-two. The precise timing, however, differs greatly from person to person.

Furthermore, only women going through spontaneous menopause—which happens when menstruation ends in midlife due to endocrine aging—will find this map applicable. Menopause strikes many women earlier in life and for various causes.

Premature or Early Menopause:

Some women have early menopause (before the age of 45) or premature menopause (before the age of 40). Primary ovarian insufficiency (POI), a disorder in which the ovaries produce insufficient amounts of reproductive hormones, accounts for 1 to 3 percent of women who experience early or premature menopause.

Some women undergo an early or premature menopause due to autoimmune or metabolic diseases, infections, or genetic factors. Nonetheless, some medical procedures and surgery are the most frequent causes of early or premature menopause. This type of menopause is known as induced menopause, and it is very different from spontaneous menopause.

Menopause Initial:

Many women experience "induced menopause," which is the cessation of ovulation brought on by either an oophorectomy, a surgical removal of the ovaries, or the ovarian function collapsing as a result of medical treatments like radiation or chemotherapy. When a woman has surgery to remove her ovaries while she is still menstruating, she will enter menopause shortly after the procedure.

Menopause can also occur earlier in life in women whose ovaries stop functioning for various medical reasons. This is referred to as medical menopause.

While medical menopause might occur over weeks or months, surgical menopause can occur extremely fast. It is noteworthy that ovulation will continue after a partial, or simple, hysterectomy, in which the uterus is removed but the ovaries remain in situ. Therefore, it won't cause an early menopause.

However, there's a chance that the ovaries' blood supply and hormone output will both decline. This could cause menopausal symptoms to appear earlier than anticipated.

MENOPAUSE: WHAT CAUSES IT?

We must first understand how hormones work prior to menopause in order to completely understand what our bodies go through during this time.

Every 28 days or so, during our reproductive years, a complex dance of hormonal feedback loops takes place. Follicle-stimulating hormone (FSH), progesterone, oestrogen (technically known as estradiol), and luteinizing hormone (LH) are the primary sex hormones involved. They fluctuate in height from the first day of your period to the day before your next one, depending on where in the menstrual cycle they occur.

The follicular phase is the initial part of the menstrual cycle. The hormones FSH and LH surge at this period to promote the development of many follicles, each of which contains an egg cell from the ovaries. Oestrogen stimulates the uterine lining to expand, just as the follicles do, giving the egg the support it needs to carry a baby.

A spike in LH leads the so-called dominant follicle to rupture, releasing the mature egg into the fallopian tube when oestrogen levels are high enough. Ovulation occurs during the middle of the cycle. At that time, pregnancy is most likely to occur.

The luteinizing phase is the second part of the cycle. If pregnancy has occurred, oestrogen and progesterone levels remain elevated to prevent the shedding of the womb lining and promote the growth of the placenta.

In the absence of pregnancy, these hormone levels fall and cause the uterus to shed its lining, which initiates menstruation. As long as these hormones are in sync, supporting and regulating each other in harmony, despite the relatively complex nature of the menstrual cycle, everything usually proceeds according to plan.

That is, unless a significant incident happens to throw off this delicate equilibrium, which is when menopause starts.

A woman's ovaries run out of eggs and begin to produce less oestrogen as she approaches menopause. Because estrogen doesn't give up quickly, this procedure isn't linear or steady.

The concentration of estrogen decreases gradually rather than all at once and can fluctuate greatly. Even so, not every woman experiences these changes. This is because the menstrual cycle causes ooestrogen levels to rise and decrease in a regular rhythm, maintaining a constant ooestrogen concentration. During the menopause transition, the duration and frequency of the menstrual cycle become more irregular, causing a wide fluctuation in the concentration of estrogen due to its dramatic peaks and troughs.

Hormone fluctuations are not limited to estrogen.

Finally, progesterone bottoms out, while FSH and LH rise in place of all the sex hormones due to a breakdown in the feedback loops that were so meticulously controlling them.

This hormonal roller coaster can cause or contribute to the seemingly random and frequently unpredictable physical and psychological side effects that many women experience throughout menopause.

SYMPTOMS

The phrase "hot and bothered" has a whole different meaning after menopause. Menopause, though commonly thought of as a single occurrence, is actually more of a syndrome with well over thirty distinct symptoms that vary depending on the individual woman. It can be confusing because some or none of these symptoms are present.

Generally speaking, with the

exception of irregular menstrual cycles that end when menopause is achieved, 10 to 15 percent of women report no changes at all. However, the great majority suffer from several hundred distinct symptom combinations.

Moreover, certain symptoms affect you from the neck down and are somatic, or of the body, while other symptoms are neurological, or originate in the brain. Notably, even though it's easy to mix up physical and mental symptoms, the menopause repertoire includes at least as many mental as physical symptoms.

For instance, a common misconception among women is that hot flashes indicate a skin condition. However, that has nothing to do with the skin. The brain is the source of hot flashes, which are a valid neurological symptom.

Let's examine these symptom categories differences in more detail.

The most common physical symptoms of menopause are numerous and profound. These encompass alterations in the frequency and pattern of menstruation, in addition to genitourinary symptoms such as dry vagina, painful sex, stress incontinence, or a hyperactive bladder. Bone-related symptoms include osteoporosis risk and bone fragility, whereas muscular changes manifest as pain, tension, joint pain, and stiffness.

Additionally, there may be changes relating to the breasts, such as edema, discomfort, and loss of fullness. But it's important to remember that menopause's less well-known physical symptoms can have a big impact on women's lives and wellbeing. These include palpitations and an irregular heartbeat, which can be extremely frightening. Changes in metabolism, weight gain, and body composition are also included, as well as digestive problems such as bloating, acid reflux, and nausea.

More symptoms include dry skin,

brittle nails, thinning hair, itching, changes in body odor, taste changes, dry or burning mouth, tinnitus, reduced hearing, noise sensitivity, and even the emergence of new allergies. It is important to take these symptoms seriously because they can be quite difficult to manage on their own. Some may even give you the impression that your body is deceiving you, give you the impression that you're losing your mind, or cause you to lose control.

However, for most women, the main cause of concern is usually the effects of menopause on the brain. Some of them, like the recognizable heat flashes discussed earlier, might be recognizable, but others might surprise you (or maybe you won't believe that the brain is also the source of them). Midlife hormonal instability can trigger changes in mood, sleep patterns, stress levels, libido, and cognitive function, in addition to body temperature. Crucially, these changes can take place without causing any heat flashes.

Furthermore, some women have neurological conditions such as dizzy spells, tiredness, headaches, and migraines.

Some, on the other hand, describe more severe symptoms, such as deep melancholy, great anxiety, panic attacks, and even what are known as electric shock feelings. The brain is where all of these symptoms begin, not the ovaries. We have made great strides in our understanding of the physiological components of menopause, but we still don't fully understand the effects of the emotional, behavioral, and cognitive changes that might occur at this time.

Regretfully, not many women—and maybe even fewer medical professionals—are fully aware of how widespread these symptoms are. Many people are also unaware of how acute, intense, and disruptive they can be.

Hot Flashes:

One thing that might not immediately grab your attention is

the gradual elimination of your period, although hot flashes are difficult to ignore. Up to 85% of women experience hot flashes, which are considered the hallmark of menopause.

The medical term "vasomotor symptoms" describes hot flashes, highlighting the dilatation or constriction of blood vessels as their cause. The chest, neck, and face typically experience this sharp spike in temperature. It's normal to perspire so hard that your skin turns red, as if you were blushing or developing a fever. If you lose too much body heat in one go, you may get chills instead. But to describe this experience as a flash is inaccurate. One moment here, the next gone? Not in a manner. It's difficult to define a flash for anyone because these menopausal symptoms might linger for up to an hour, at least. Once you have one, they not only take time to go away but also have the ability to remain in your life for a considerable amount of time.

Hot flashes often last three to five years for women, but many can last ten years or more. It's also possible that lifestyle, culture, and ethnicity play a part.

For unknown reasons, Asian women report fewer hot flashes than their Caucasian counterparts, while African American and Afro-diasporic women typically have more frequent and severe hot flashes.

Hot flashes, which can range from uncomfortable to excruciating, are particularly painful when they happen at night. In this context, they use the nickname "night sweats."

Most people don't notice the difference until they really experience it. Medical textbooks define night sweats as recurrent bouts of intense perspiration while you sleep—enough to drench your sheets or nightgowns. But experiencing night sweats in real life is a very different story. Night sweats are better characterized by the ladies, who experience them as akin to a five-alarm fire—like throwing off the covers and jumping into an Arctic cold shower.

These occurrences can be extremely crippling, especially if they frequently happen—sometimes more than twice or three times per night. This also helps to explain the reputation of menopausal women as being emotionally unstable. Feeling depressed seems inevitable when you're unable to have a good night's sleep for months or even years at a time, and you're not just dealing with flashbacks but also clinical-level sleep deprivation.

Emotional Changes"

Mood swings and depression symptoms during perimenopause and in the years following the last menstrual cycle affect about 20 percent of all women. Menopause is a powerful inducer of the blues, even though it does not directly cause sadness.

Hormone changes can cause mood fluctuations that impair your ability to handle situations you would normally be able to handle.

Furthermore, some women—particularly those who have already had significant depression—may experience real depressive episodes as a result of these hormone dips. In certain situations, symptoms could resurface as the menopause progresses.

Furthermore, during the perimenopause, some women who have never experienced depression in their lives may realize that it is something they are struggling with for the first time.

Emotional changes such as anger, anxiety, and a decreased capacity to handle day-to-day difficulties frequently accompany menopause. Emotional flatness, difficulty becoming motivated, or a sense of overwhelm can also occur, along with feelings of melancholy, exhaustion, lack of motivation, and difficulty concentrating. Crying or letting out other emotions can happen more frequently, more intensely, or even seemingly out of the blue.

Although less common, some women even report experiencing panic attacks, and others describe feeling absolutely furious—all of which can easily contribute to the reputation of the crazy, evil, and dangerous menopausal woman.

This moodiness might not be all that mysterious when you consider what a life filled with constant heat flashes can be like. However, hot flashes and other symptoms are not always present in menopausal depression.

Consult a healthcare professional if you are experiencing mood swings or depressive symptoms. They can help diagnose if your feelings of depression, anxiety, or melancholy are due to menopause or whether you have clinical depression of another kind. Given that the symptoms of menopausal depression and major depression overlap, it's important to get to the root of the issue and seek the right treatment.

The good news is that there are treatments for mood swings. If the ups and downs of perimenopause affect your relationships or regular daily activities, consult your doctor about your options. Thankfully, there are a range of treatments available, including lifestyle modifications like a specially designed diet and exercise regimen, as well as menopause hormone therapy and/or antidepressants.

Remember that after menopause, hormones tend to level out, and mood swings also tend to stop.

Sleepless Nights:

Although less well-known, poor sleep quality and sleep disruptions are very common throughout this stage of life. Menopause can fuel the fire, turning what would have been a progressive process into a quick kick toward sleep deprivation, even if sleep quality naturally falls with age.
Night sweats, in particular, cause you to wake up in the middle of the night, which can lead to poor sleep if you're lucky or full-blown insomnia if you're not.

Poor sleep undoubtedly affects a person's mood and mental stability, as previously mentioned. Chronic sleep problems can lead to fatigue and cognitive fog in addition to low mood, anxiety, and possibly depression. Your brain is further confused by lower estrogen levels, which makes it harder for you to cope with stress in the first place.

Resting our active minds is necessary for the long term, since sleep is critical for memory formation, reducing the risk of cognitive impairment in old age, and quelling inflammation. This is even more problematic. For this reason, managing sleep issues that arise during the menopause transition is crucial.
Perimenopausal and postmenopausal women report greater sleep problems than any other group in the human population, which may come as no surprise.

Additionally, they report spin-off issues, including worry, tension, cognitive fog, and depressive symptoms, more frequently than normal people. The good news is that although many women experience severe sleep difficulties during perimenopause, many eventually establish a new normal, and a few years after entering the postmenopausal stage, their sleep quality improves rather quickly. But an equal number still struggle with insufficient sleep and, frequently, insomnia.

Worse, compared to premenopausal women, postmenopausal women are two to three times more likely to experience new sleep issues, including sleep apnea. Despite the general belief that this illness primarily affects men, women become more susceptible after menopause, likely due to changes in muscle tone.

Sleep apnea, a chronic breathing condition, causes recurrent mid-sleep breathing stops. This typically results from either a suppressed brain signal to initiate a breath or a partial or complete obstruction (or collapse) of the upper airway, which frequently affects the base of the tongue and the soft palate. These occurrences, which can occasionally happen hundreds of times a night and last ten seconds or more, seriously disturb sleep. The prevalence of sleep apnea is higher than you may imagine.

The National Sleep Foundation reports that sleep apnea may affect up to 20% of people, despite the fact that up to 85% of those affected are unaware of their condition. This appears to be especially true for women for two reasons. First off, rather than sleep apnea, a lot of women mistakenly believe that stress, overwork, or menopause are the cause of symptoms and effects of sleep problems, such as daytime exhaustion. Second, women frequently have more mild sleep apnea symptoms than men. Therefore, women are less likely to undergo sleep apnea evaluations, leading to a delay in diagnosis and treatment.

Given the significance of sleep for your physical and emotional health,

if you're concerned that your sleep issues could stem from sleep apnea, menopause, or a combination of both, I strongly recommend undergoing a thorough sleep evaluation. There are treatments for sleep apnea, and these frequently involve changing one's lifestyle and using a breathing aid at night, like a continuous positive airway pressure (CPAP) machine. Menopause-related sleep difficulties are crucial to treat.

Memory Loss:

Brain fog is something many women don't expect to accompany sweating and restless nights. Few things are more unsettling than experiencing a decline in memory or a brain that no longer functions as the sharp and helpful tool it once was. Though not a medical word, "brain fog" accurately characterizes the foggy thinking, fuzzy mental state, and trouble processing information that frequently follow menopause.

The best way to describe this phenomenon is probably to feel as though you are covered in cotton wool and that it is difficult to focus on daily tasks that now take more time, effort, and concentration, or to take in and remember information. The most frequent complaints are things like losing focus when working on a mental activity, forgetting why you entered a room, and having trouble remembering words and familiar names.

More than 60% of all perimenopausal and postmenopausal women have brain fog, according to current statistics. Because of how distinct the experience is, it may make one feel less productive, particularly when memory gaps occur. It's crucial to understand that perimenopause can cause a jump in forgetfulness, which can exacerbate worries about going insane and developing early-stage dementia. In other words, millions of young, healthy women experience a sense of unpredictability. They feel as though their bodies, brains, and doctors have failed them, unaware that the symptoms they are experiencing are actually signs of menopause.

That's the bad news. The good news is that menopausal fog or forgetfulness does not always indicate the onset of dementia. As a field specialist, I want to reassure everyone that there is a significant difference between feeling like your mental capacity is declining and actually being clinically impaired. The power surges and sputters you're experiencing don't necessarily indicate that the lights are going out, even though the aforementioned symptoms may be unbearable and test your patience to the limit. In fact, in the medical community, brain fog is known as subjective cognitive decline, or mental tiredness.

Here, "subjective" is crucial. This definition states that patients are "aware of a decline from a previous level of cognitive functioning, in the absence of objective impairment," when it comes to midlife women. To put it another way, even if you think that your performance falls short of your typical standards—

which are based on a subjective assessment—it's likely that your performance is objectively within the relevant reference range or comparable to that of other individuals in your age group.

Since two-thirds of Alzheimer's patients are female, it is clear that women are not immune to cognitive decline. Some people may have a decline in cognitive function during menopause, which could eventually lead to a dementia diagnosis. Similarly, in our brain imaging studies, some women see less change in their brain energy during menopause, while others experience more severe impairments in other critical functions. This is definitely a warning sign for an increased chance of dementia in later life.

All of this implies that women who are concerned about brain fog in their middle years should take this knowledge seriously and take excellent care of their brains both during and after menopause.

Alzheimer's disease causes foggy thinking, which also manifests as trouble remembering things, finding the correct words, and organizing thoughts. Therefore, how can we differentiate between them?

Menopause-related memory changes typically don't interfere too much with your everyday life to the point where they are functionally incapacitating. Additionally, they either resolve over time or stay stable. Alzheimer's is a degenerative disease that deteriorates over time and affects your capacity to function and take care of yourself, unlike menopausal fog. In this context, dementia is defined as forgetting the purposes for which one has money, not that one has money.

If your menopausal cognitive problems are significantly interfering with your everyday life and don't seem to get better on their own, medication, or lifestyle changes, you may want to consult a neuropsychologist or a neurologist. For instance, if your severe concerns persist three to four years after menopause, now would be an ideal moment to undergo testing, if only to ensure your peace of mind. Additionally, I would advise enrolling in a program that prevents Alzheimer's.

MENOPAUSE AND NUTRITION

In our culture, dieting is more important than self-nourishment when it comes to losing weight. Without a doubt, this is absolutely wrong! Choosing carefully what we put in our mouths is essential for maintaining our health and wellbeing throughout our lives.

Nutrition is defined as the consumption of food and how the body uses it for energy production, growth, repair, and general health maintenance. To support physiological processes and avoid nutritional deficits, it entails consuming macronutrients (proteins, fats, and carbohydrates) and micronutrients (vitamins and minerals) in the proper amounts.

Macronutrients:

- **Carbohydrates:** Carbohydrates are the body's primary energy source. Whole grains, fruits, vegetables, and legumes include complex carbs, which improve digestive health and control blood sugar levels in addition to providing long-lasting energy and dietary fiber.

- **Proteins:** Immune system performance, muscular growth, and tissue healing all depend on proteins. Lean protein sources —fish, chicken, tofu, lentils, and low-fat dairy—offer the amino acids required to sustain metabolic health and preserve muscle mass. In order to maintain muscle strength and metabolic efficiency during menopause and possibly avoid weight gain and metabolic disorders, an adequate protein intake is critical.

- **Fats:** Good fats play a critical role in hormone production, cognitive function, and fat-soluble vitamin absorption.

Olive oil, avocados, nuts, seeds, and fatty fish are good sources of monounsaturated and polyunsaturated fats that can lower cholesterol, reduce inflammation, and improve cardiovascular health. Limiting processed foods, fried foods, and fatty meats that contain trans and saturated fats can help lower the risk of heart disease and other chronic illnesses.

Micronutrients:

- **Vitamins:** Vitamins are essential for several physiological functions, including immune system performance, energy metabolism, and bone health. Vitamin B complex, which helps regulate mood and energy levels, and vitamin D, which promotes the immune system and bone health, are important vitamins for managing menopause. Vitamins are abundant in fruits, vegetables, whole grains, and fortified diets.

- **Minerals:** Minerals are essential for hormone balance, muscle contraction, and bone health. During menopause, calcium, magnesium, and phosphorus are especially crucial for preserving bone density and averting osteoporosis. Rich sources of minerals include leafy greens, dairy products, nuts, seeds, and legumes.

- **Phytonutrients:** Plant-based diets contain bioactive substances called phytonutrients that have anti-inflammatory, antioxidant, and other health-promoting qualities. Phytoestrogens, which are phytonutrients with weak estrogenic activities like lignans and isoflavones, may lessen menopausal symptoms like hot flashes and dry vaginas. Phytoestrogens are abundant in whole grains, legumes, flaxseeds, and chickpeas.

The Role of Diet in Menopause Management

The role of nutrition in menopause treatment includes the use of dietary techniques to maintain general health, lessen menopausal symptoms, lower the risk of long-term consequences, and enhance wellbeing both during and after the menopausal transition.

This all-encompassing strategy entails understanding the unique nutritional requirements and difficulties that women encounter during menopause and customizing dietary interventions to target specific issues and objectives.

Mitigating Menopausal Symptoms:

In order to mitigate common menopausal symptoms like mood swings, vaginal dryness, hot flashes, and sleep difficulties, nutrition is essential. Specific nutrients and dietary components such as phytoestrogens, omega-3 fatty acids, complex carbohydrates, and vitamins have demonstrated their ability to alleviate these symptoms. Researchers have also found these components to modify hormone levels, stabilize mood, maintain vaginal health, and improve sleep quality.

Supporting Bone Health:

During menopause, a drop in estrogen levels leads to a decrease in bone density and an increased risk of osteoporosis. Sustaining bone health and avoiding fractures during and after menopause requires an adequate intake of calcium, vitamin D, magnesium, and other minerals that promote the health of the bones. A diet high in calcium-rich meals, fortified foods, leafy greens, and vitamin D sources is one way to optimize bone health.

Managing Weight and Metabolism:

Menopause-related hormonal changes can interfere with metabolism and make women more likely to gain weight, particularly around the abdomen. During menopause, a healthy, well-balanced diet high in fiber, lean proteins, and healthy fats can promote metabolic health, control appetite, and help with weight management.

Prioritize portion control, thoughtful eating, and regular

exercise to aid in weight management.

Promoting Heart Health:

Hormonal changes and age-related variables contribute to an increased risk of cardiovascular disease after menopause.
Diet can partially mitigate cardiovascular risk factors such as inflammation, high blood pressure, and excessive cholesterol. Implementing a heart-healthy diet full of fruits, vegetables, whole grains, lean meats, and healthy fats can help maintain cardiovascular health and lower the risk of heart disease both during and after menopause.

Enhancing Overall Well-being:

Not only can diet address some symptoms and health issues associated with menopause, but it also enhances general health and quality of life during this time. Essential nutrients, antioxidants, and phytonutrients that support immune system function, energy levels, cognitive function, and skin health can be found in a balanced and varied diet. Keeping hydrated, drinking enough water, and eating high-water content meals are also critical for preserving general health throughout menopause.

Personalized Approach:

It is imperative to acknowledge that women may exhibit distinct nutrition requirements and reactions to dietary interventions, contingent upon variables such as age, body composition, metabolism, health state, and individual preferences.
Consequently, it is crucial to treat menopause through a personalized approach to nutrition. A healthcare professional or registered dietitian can assist in developing personalized nutrition regimens that fit each person's needs, address specific issues, and improve health outcomes both during and after menopause.

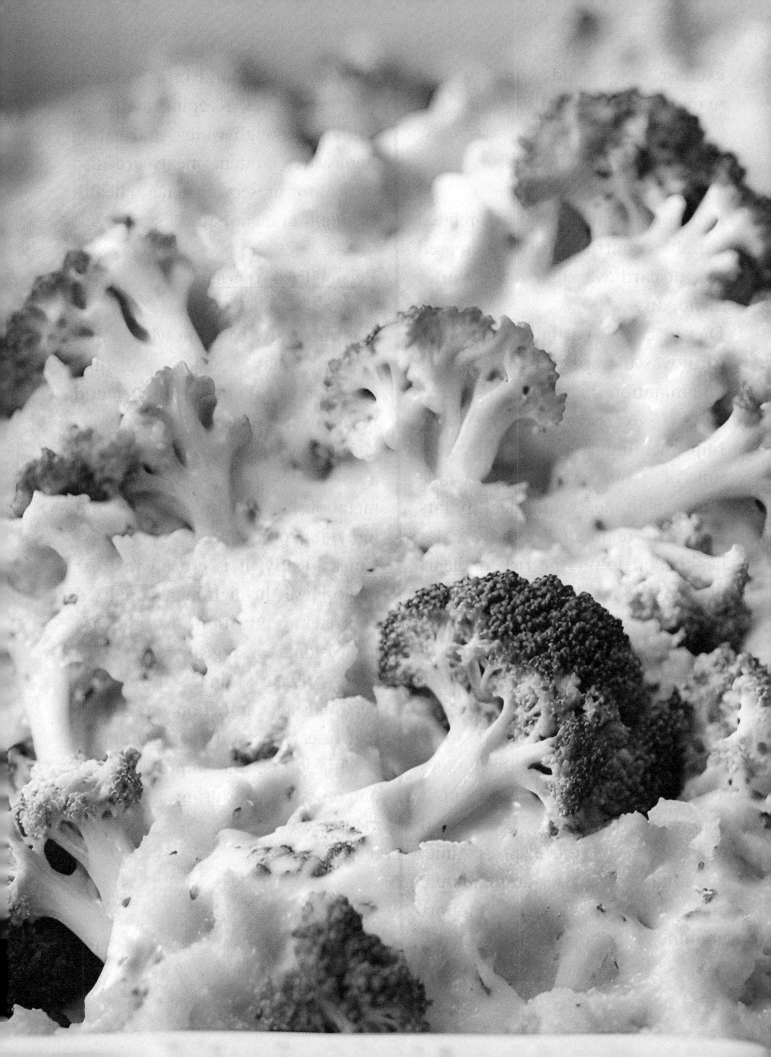

LOADED HUMUS BOWL

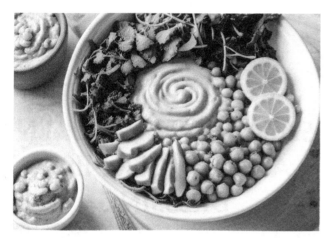

Servings: 4

Ingredients

Hummus

- 4 garlic cloves, divided
- 1 large lemon, juiced
- One 14.5-ounce can chickpeas, drained and rinsed
- ½ teaspoon baking soda
- ⅓ cup tahini
- Sea salt

Tempeh and greens

- 2 tablespoons olive oil
- 12 ounces tempeh, crumbled
- 1 teaspoon sea salt
- 1 teaspoon freshly ground black pepper
- 1 teaspoon cumin
- ½ teaspoon coriander
- ½ teaspoon cayenne pepper
- 4 cups spinach or baby kale

Toppings

- ½ cup pitted Castelvetrano olives, chopped
- ½ red onion, diced
- 1 cup cherry tomatoes, halved
- ¼ cup roasted pumpkin seeds
- Extra-virgin olive oil Sumac, cumin, or paprika

Directions:

- Using the flat side of your knife, crush two of the garlic cloves.
- Transfer them to a little bowl and pour the lemon juice over them. While you cook the chickpeas, set aside the raw garlic to let it soften in the acidic juice.
- In a large saucepan, combine the chickpeas, ½ teaspoon baking soda, and the remaining 2 garlic cloves.
- Pour in some water, cover, and cook until it boils. Lower the heat to medium and simmer the mixture until the chickpeas become so tender that their skins are beginning to peel, around 25 to 30 minutes.
- After cooking the chickpeas and garlic, strain them and place them in a food processor.

- Stir in the tahini and lemon juice along with the garlic. After blending until smooth, carefully pour in enough filtered water to the food processor while it's operating to assist transform the texture from slightly gritty to the ideal velvety consistency. (It should only require a few tablespoons for this.)
- After adding sea salt to taste, leave aside and get the tempeh and vegetables ready.
- In a big skillet set over medium-high heat, warm the olive oil. Add the following five ingredients together with the crumbled tempeh.
- Add the greens and stir-fry the tempeh for a few minutes until it starts to get crispy and brown around the edges.
- Simmer the greens for a further one to two minutes, or until they begin to gently wilt.
- Using the back of a spoon, divide the hummus among 4 bowls, making sure to leave an even, wavy layer.
- Spoon the greens and tempeh evenly among the bowls, then garnish with the olives, onions, tomatoes, and pumpkin seeds for each serving.
- Add a final flourish of sumac and a small spray of olive oil to each bowl.

BRUSSEL SPROUT SALAD WITH CHICKEN AND GINGER MISO DRESSING

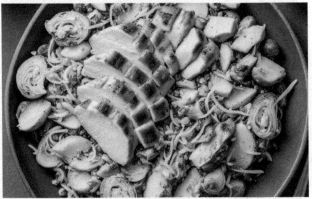

Servings: 4
Ingredients
Chicken

- 2 boneless, skinless chicken breasts, halved
- 1 teaspoon sea salt
- 1 teaspoon freshly ground black pepper
- 1 teaspoon garlic powder
- ½ teaspoon onion powder
- 2 tablespoons avocado oil

Salad

- 4 cups brussels sprouts, trimmed and shaved

- 4 scallions, roots trimmed, sliced thin
- ¼ cup slivered almonds
- 2 tablespoons whole flaxseeds
- 2 tablespoons toasted sesame seeds

Dressing
- ¼ cup avocado oil
- 1 tablespoon toasted sesame oil
- 3 tablespoons rice vinegar
- 3 tablespoons coconut aminos 1 tablespoon freshly grated ginger
- 2 teaspoons white miso paste
- 1 garlic clove, grated

Directions:
- Use salt, pepper, onion powder, and garlic powder to season the chicken on all sides.
- In a big skillet, warm the avocado oil over medium-high heat. When the oil is hot, add the chicken and cook it for five to six minutes on each side, or until it is cooked through and golden. Take off the heat and place aside.
- All the salad components should be combined in a big bowl.
- In a medium-sized bowl, add all the dressing ingredients and

- whisk to properly blend.
- Add the chicken to the dish of Brussels sprout salad after chopping it up into bite-sized pieces. Toss with the dressing and serve.

SHAKSHUKA WITH PICKLED ONIONS AND AVOCADO

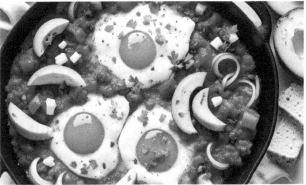

Servings: 4

Ingredients
- 2 tablespoons olive oil
- 1 yellow onion, peeled and diced
- 4 garlic cloves, minced
- 1 red bell pepper, seeded and diced
- 3 tablespoons tomato paste
- 2 tablespoons harissa
- 1 teaspoon sea salt
- 1 teaspoon freshly ground black pepper
- 1 teaspoon cumin
- ½ teaspoon paprika

- One 28-ounce can crush tomatoes
- 2 cups baby kale
- 8 eggs
- 1 large avocado, pitted, scooped out of the skin, and sliced
- 1 cup pickled red onion
- ¼ cup chopped cilantro

Directions:

- Over medium-high heat, pour the olive oil into a large skillet.
- Add the onion and sauté, stirring, for approximately 2 minutes, or until it begins to turn translucent.
- Next, add the bell pepper and garlic.
- Stir in the harissa, tomato paste, cumin, paprika, salt, and pepper after cooking for an additional two minutes. Cook, stirring, until the mixture takes on a fragrant aroma.
- After adding the crushed tomatoes, reduce the heat if the sauce begins to bubble or sputter. After 20 minutes of simmering, the mixture will gradually thicken.
- Cook the kale until it wilts after adding it. One egg at a time,

carefully add them in, being careful to preserve the yolks.

- Once the eggs are set and the yolks are cooked to your desired doneness, cover the pan and continue cooking for an additional five to six minutes.
- Top the shakshuka with the pickled onion, avocado, and cilantro and serve.

KIMCHI SALAD WITH CRISPY CHICKPEAS

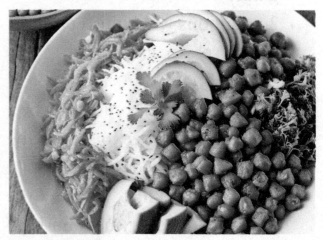

Servings: 4

Ingredients

Chickpeas

- 2 tablespoons olive oil
- One 14.5-ounce can chickpeas, drained and rinsed
- ½ teaspoon sea salt
- ½ teaspoon garlic powder
- ½ teaspoon onion powder
- ½ teaspoon turmeric
- ½ teaspoon cumin

Dressing

- ¼ cup avocado oil
- 3 tablespoons rice vinegar
- 3 tablespoons coconut aminos
- 1 garlic clove, grated
- Sea salt
- Freshly ground black pepper

Salad

- 1 cup kimchi, drained and chopped
- 1 head of romaine lettuce, trimmed and chopped
- 2 cups baby spinach
- 8 radishes, trimmed and thinly sliced
- 2 tablespoons hemp seeds
- 2 tablespoons sesame seeds

Directions:

- Over medium-high heat, warm the olive oil in a large skillet. Fill the skillet with the chickpeas.
- In a small bowl, mix together the salt, cumin, turmeric, onion powder, and garlic powder. Over the chickpeas, spread the spice mixture.
- Cook, stirring to ensure that the spices are uniformly distributed, until the chickpeas begin to crackle and become brown around the edges. Take off the heat and place aside.

- In a small bowl, mix together the avocado oil, vinegar, coconut aminos, and garlic. Add salt and pepper to taste and whisk to combine the dressing.
- Toss the salad ingredients together in a large bowl. After adding the dressing and scattering the crunchy chickpeas over the salad, stir and serve.

ALMOND CHICKEN TENDERS AND SAUERKRAUT SLAW

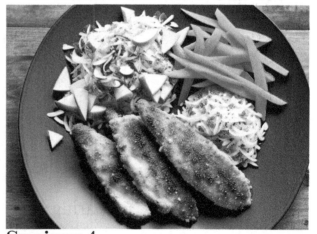

Servings: 4

Ingredients

Slaw

- 2 cups sauerkraut, drained
- 2 celery stalks, thinly sliced
- 1 large Granny Smith apple, cored, halved, and thinly sliced

- ¼ cup apple cider vinegar
- ¼ cup roasted pumpkin seeds, hemp seeds, or flaxseeds
- 2 tablespoons avocado oil

Chicken

- ½ cup almond meal
- 3 tablespoons nutritional yeast
- 1½ teaspoons sea salt
- 1 teaspoon freshly ground black pepper
- 1 teaspoon paprika
- 1 teaspoon garlic powder
- ½ teaspoon onion powder
- 1 egg
- ½ cup unsweetened almond milk
- 1 pound chicken tenderloins
- 2 tablespoons avocado oil

Directions:

- Set oven temperature to 400°F.
- Put parchment paper on one baking sheet and set it aside.
- In a large bowl, add all the slaw ingredients and toss to combine them. While preparing the tenders, season to taste with salt, cover, and store in the refrigerator.
- In a large shallow bowl or pie plate, combine the almond meal, yeast, salt, pepper, paprika, garlic powder, and onion powder.
- In another wide-brimmed dish, whisk together the egg and almond milk.
- Install a station for dredging. Gently press and roll the chicken tender in the almond meal coating after dipping it on both sides in the egg mixture.
- Once completely coated, place the chicken on the baking sheet that has been prepared. Continue until you have covered every tender.
- Apply a little coating of oil onto the tenderloins' surface. Bake for thirty to forty minutes after placing in the oven.
- Together with a heaping of the slaw, serve the chicken tenders.

GARLIC-GINGER TEMPEH AND BROCCOLI OVER QUINOA

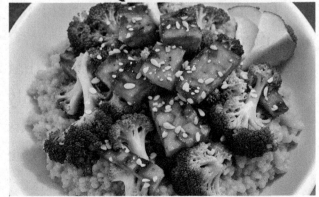

Servings: 4

Ingredients

- 6 garlic cloves, minced
- 2 tablespoons freshly grated ginger
- 2 tablespoons toasted sesame oil
- ⅓ cup coconut aminos
- 1 large lemon, juiced and zested 2 tablespoons avocado oil
- 12 ounces tempeh, cut into thin strips or crumbled
- 2 cups broccoli florets
- Sea salt
- Freshly ground pepper
- 1 cup quinoa, prepared according to the package instructions
- 1½ cups kimchi

Directions:

- Mix the first five ingredients together in a medium-sized bowl.Mix thoroughly and reserve.
- Over medium-high heat, warm the oil in a big skillet. After adding the tempeh and cooking it until the edges start to turn golden brown, add the broccoli.
- After adding salt and pepper to taste, simmer for approximately four minutes.
- Pour in the garlic-ginger combination and turn the heat down to medium.
- Simmer until the broccoli is fork-tender and the sauce has thickened. Serve with a serving of kimchi over the cooked quinoa.

KIMCHI STEW WITH TOFU

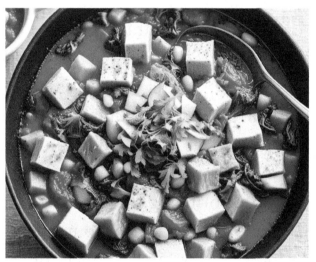

Servings: 4

Ingredients

- 2 tablespoons avocado oil
- 1 yellow onion, diced
- 6 garlic cloves, minced
- 3 cups kimchi, chopped
- 2 tablespoons chili paste
- 5 cups vegetable broth
- 1 15 ounce can cannellini or navy beans, drained and rinsed
- Sea salt
- Freshly ground black pepper

- 12 ounces extra-firm tofu, cubed
- 4 scallions, thinly sliced
- ¼ cup cilantro, chopped
- Toasted sesame oil

Directions:

- In a big pot, warm the avocado oil over medium-high heat. Cook the onion and garlic together for two to three minutes, or until the onion begins to turn translucent.
- Stir in the chili paste and kimchi. After a minute of stirring and cooking, add the broth, the beans, and salt and pepper to taste.
- After bringing the mixture to a boil, lower the heat to medium-low, cover, and simmer for 20 minutes.
- Cook the tofu for an additional fifteen minutes in the pot with a lid on.
- Reduce the heat to a simmer if the stew is boiling when the tofu is added.
- Add the cilantro, scallions, and a dab of toasted sesame oil to the stew before serving.

PROSCIUTTO, SPINACH, AND ASPARAGUS FRITTATA

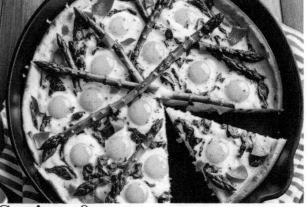

Servings: 8

Ingredients

- 8 eggs
- ½ cup unsweetened almond milk
- ⅓ cup nutritional yeast
- 1 teaspoon sea salt
- 1 teaspoon freshly ground black pepper
- 2 tablespoons ghee
- 1 large shallot, finely diced
- 3 garlic cloves, minced
- 4 ounces prosciutto, chopped
- 1 pound asparagus, woody ends removed, cut into 2 to 3-inch pieces
- 3 cups spinach

Directions:

- Set oven temperature to 350°F.
- Over medium-high heat, preheat a sizable cast-iron pan

(or other oven-safe pan).

- In a medium bowl, mix together the eggs, almond milk, yeast, salt, and pepper.
- After fully whisking, set aside.
- Add the ghee to the pan once it's heated.
- Add the garlic and shallot after allowing the ghee to melt. Add the prosciutto and cook for 1 to 2 minutes, or until the shallot begins to turn translucent. Simmer for a further three to four minutes. When the prosciutto begins to crisp and turn golden, add the asparagus.
- Add the spinach and cook for a few minutes, or until the spinach wilts, after the asparagus has turned a vibrant green color.
- Over the sautéed vegetables, pour the egg mixture. Simmer for 3 to 4 minutes, or until the frittata's bottom starts to set. After placing the frittata in the oven, bake it for 15 minutes, or until the eggs are set in the middle.
- Serve the frittata by cutting it like a pie.

BRATS WITH SAUTÉED APPLES AND ONIONS (SERVE WITH SAUERKRAUT)

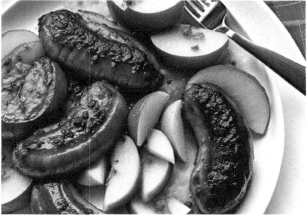

Servings: 4

Ingredients

- 2 tablespoons olive oil
- 1-pound brats, cut into medallions
- 1 large onion, halved and thinly sliced
- 2 Granny Smith apples, cored, peeled, and thinly sliced
- ¼ cup apple cider vinegar
- ¼ cup seeds such as flax, pumpkin, hemp, or a combo of all 3
- 1 teaspoon smoked paprika
- Sea salt
- Freshly ground black pepper
- 1½ cups sauerkraut

Directions:

- In a big skillet set over

- medium-high heat, warm the olive oil. Stirring to ensure even searing, add the brats and cook for approximately two minutes. Toss the onion.
- Cook the onion for a further five to six minutes, or until it is tender and translucent—almost caramelized. Taste and adjust the seasoning with salt and pepper after adding the apples, vinegar, seeds, and paprika.
- Simmer for a few more minutes, or until the liquid has reduced by more than half and the apples are soft.
- Present alongside a dollop of sauerkraut.

COCONUT AND KALE LENTIL SOUP

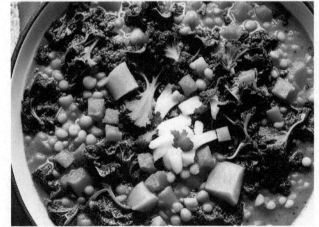

Servings: 4
Ingredients
- 1 cup unsweetened shredded coconut
- 2 tablespoons avocado oil
- 1 yellow onion, diced
- 6 garlic cloves, minced
- 2 tablespoons freshly grated ginger
- 2 tablespoons red curry paste
- 1 cup red split lentils
- 5 cups vegetable broth
- 1 teaspoon salt
- 1 teaspoon freshly ground black pepper
- One 14.5-ounce can full-fat coconut milk
- 4 cups kale, stems removed, chopped
- ¼ cup seeds of your choosing (pumpkin, flax, hemp)

Directions:
- Turn the heat up to medium-high in a big pot. When the saucepan is hot, pour in the coconut shreds.
- Stirring constantly, dry roast the coconut in the pot until it begins to take on a light golden-brown color. As soon as possible, move the toasted coconut to a medium-sized bowl and reserve.
- Transfer the saucepan back to the burner and pour in the

- avocado oil.
- Add the onion and cook for 2 to 3 minutes, or until it begins to become translucent.
- Next, add the ginger and garlic. Add the red curry paste and stir; cook for just a minute or so.
- Stir the mixture constantly over the fire until it starts to smell pleasant.
- Add the toasted coconut that was set aside, the lentils, the broth, salt, and pepper.
- Following a boil, lower the heat to medium-low, cover the pot, and simmer the mixture for 25 to 30 minutes, or until the lentils are soft and well cooked.
- A few minutes prior to serving, mix in the kale and coconut milk.
- Continue heating the soup until the kale begins to wilt. Add extra salt and pepper to taste, then top the soup with a sprinkling of seeds and serve.

PULLED PORK IN BONE BROTH

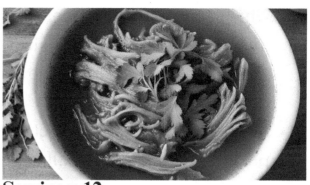

Servings: 12
Ingredients
- 1 teaspoon salt (or to taste)
- ½ teaspoon pepper (or to taste)
- 6 pounds pork shoulder
- 8 cups Basic Beef Bone Broth
- Juice of 2 lemons
- 2 tablespoons ground cumin
- 3 to 4 bay leaves
- 2 tablespoons ground herbes de Provence
- ½ teaspoon cayenne pepper
- ¼ cup chopped cilantro
- 1 medium organic yellow onion, cored
- 1 teaspoon arrowroot powder

Directions:
- There exist four methods for braising. The quickest to slowest techniques are as follows:
- 1 hour for pressure cooking
- 3–4 hours on the stovetop
- 4–8 hours in the oven
- 4–8 hours for slow cooking.
- The slow cooker method, for

- which these instructions are intended, takes the least amount of time and should hold six or more quarts.
- Generously season the entire pork shoulder with salt and pepper.
- Set a big sauté or frying pan over medium-high heat. Put the meat in the pan and sear it until it turns a light golden brown on all sides.
- This is a crucial stage since it involves two processes that will contribute to the final dish's deliciousness: flavor creation and moisture retention. The flavor of all the crispy bits will permeate your braising liquid.
- Before adding the ingredients to the slow cooker, bring the Basic Beef Bone Broth, lemon juice, and spices to a boil.
- Cook on low for eight hours after adding the liquids, pork, and onion to the slow cooker. Observe that the liquid ought to merely envelop the meat.
- After cooking, you can reserve some of the Basic Beef Bone Broth to include with the shredded beef; but, before doing so, you should slightly thicken it with arrowroot powder.
- To achieve this, add a teaspoon of arrowroot powder to a small amount of boiling liquid at a time, blend well, and then return the mixture to the sauce-making liquid you set aside.
- Using two forks, remove the meat from the slow cooker, shred it, and then stir in the thickened sauce.

BACON, AVOCADO, EGG

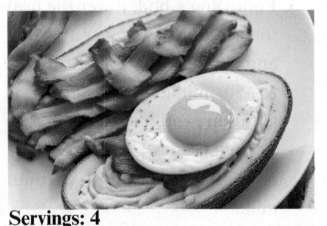

Servings: 4
Ingredients
- 4 large avocados
- 1 teaspoon salt
- ¼ cup raw apple cider vinegar
- 4 large free-range chicken or duck eggs
- 16 slices hormone-free bacon

Directions:
- Halve the avocados and take out the seeds. To create space

- for the poached egg that will go within, gently scoop off a small quantity of avocado from the middle.
- Peel the avocado skin carefully. Put aside.
- Add three to four inches of water to a saucepan.
- Bring the mixture to a boil after adding the apple cider vinegar and ½ teaspoon of salt. Give eggs a five-minute poach.
- Gently slide one poached egg into one avocado half, then cover the opening with the other half. Wrap around 4 bacon slices around each avocado.
- Heat a pan with a curve on high heat. Sear the bacon on the avocado's exterior, turning it over carefully, until it's crispy and evenly golden brown.
- A nice approach to sear the curved parts of an avocado is to lean it along the edge of a curved pan. The avocado and the egg within will be held together by the crisp bacon, which forms a shell as it cooks.
- Serve right away.

Tip:
- When poaching, the acid from the vinegar in the water keeps the egg together.
- The secret to searing the avocado wrapped in bacon is high heat—it must get hot quickly or the texture of the soft avocado underneath will suffer.
- This dish tastes great served with a mixed green salad with sliced heirloom tomatoes, chopped parsley, and crumbled feta cheese.

ROASTED LEG OF LAMB

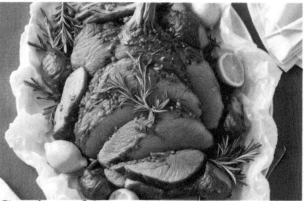

Servings: 20
Ingredients
- 5 pounds boneless leg of lamb
- 8 fresh rosemary sprigs
- Zest and juice of 2 lemons
- 1 tablespoon minced garlic
- ¼ cup avocado oil
- 2 teaspoons salt

- 1 teaspoon ground pepper
- Two 10-gallon clear plastic garbage bags

Directions:

- Put all the materials into two 10-gallon transparent plastic waste bags (for added strength).
- When adding the rosemary sprigs, proceed with additional caution to ensure they do not pierce the plastic. To ensure that the entire leg of lamb is marinated, make sure all the air is out of the bags and tie a knot at the top.
- To marinate for 4 hours or up to 2 days, place the lamb in a basin or on a plate (only in case it leaks).
- Grill the lamb for 45 minutes, or until it's cooked through, over medium heat. Alternately, cook it for 45 minutes at 375°F in the oven after starting it on the grill to obtain color.

ROASTED CHICKEN

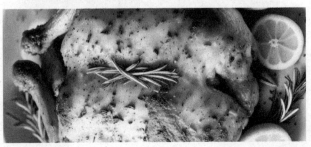

Servings: 4

Ingredients

- 1 whole chicken
- 3 lemons, sliced
- 5 fresh rosemary sprigs
- 1 teaspoon sea salt
- ½ teaspoon ground pepper
- Dash of paprika

Directions:

- Set oven temperature to 375°F.
- Cover a roasting pan with parchment paper, making sure to tuck the edges in between the drip pan.
- Take off the spine and butterfly your chicken. Either a knife or a set of robust kitchen shears would work for this.
- By taking away the spine, you may make the chicken flatter on the roasting pan, which will allow it to cook faster and more evenly while maintaining its crispy outer and juicy within.
- Line the bottom of the roasting pan with parchment paper and make a bed of lemon slices and rosemary sprigs.
- On top of the lemons and rosemary, arrange the chicken. Add the paprika, pepper, and salt on top.
- Bake for 45 to 55 minutes, or

- until the chicken's juices are clear.

KETOBIOTIC WAFFLES

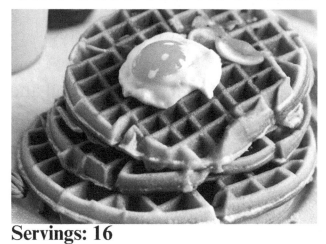

Servings: 16

Ingredients

- 3 cups blanched almond flour
- ¼ cup shredded coconut, unsweetened
- 1 teaspoon baking powder
- ¼ teaspoon sea salt
- ½ teaspoon ground cinnamon
- ⅔ cup coconut milk
- ¼ cup maple syrup
- 2 teaspoons vanilla extract
- 5 free-range eggs, yolks and whites separated
- ⅓ cup grass-fed butter, softened
- For chocolate waffles, add ¼ cup raw cacao powder.

Directions:

- Waffle irons should be turned on at the desired setting.
- In a medium bowl, combine all the dry ingredients and stir until well combined.
  - In a sizable bowl, cream the butter, egg yolks, maple syrup, vanilla, and coconut milk.
  - In another medium-sized dish, beat the egg whites until soft peaks form.
  - Fold the egg whites gently into the large bowl's egg-yolk mixture.
  - Till they are completely combined, gently mix the dry ingredients into the creamed liquid ingredients.
  - Place a dollop of batter in the center of the waffle square using a 2-ounce ladle.
  - Cook for the recommended amount of time on the waffle iron (around 4 minutes). Cook the waffle batter until it is all utilized.

CRUSTLESS QUICHE

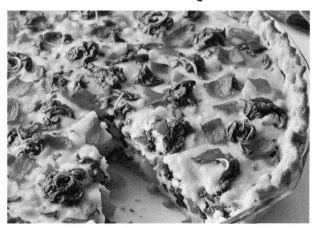

Servings: 8
Ingredients

- 1 cup diced onion, sautéed until clear
- 3 cups (total) of whatever you have in your kitchen, such as:
- 1 cup frozen organic spinach, thawed, squeezed, finely diced
- 1 cup diced bacon, cooked
- 1 cup diced (½-inch cubes) butternut squash
- 1 cup diced roasted red bell peppers
- 3 cups (total) of whatever cheese you have, such as:
- 1½ cups shredded goat cheddar cheese
- 1½ cups shredded raw Parmesan cheese
- 8 large free-range eggs, beaten
- ½ teaspoon salt
- ½ teaspoon pepper
- 1 teaspoon of the herb of your choice (mine is herbes de Provence)

Directions:

- Set oven temperature to 350°F.
- Grease a baking dish that is 8 inches square with butter.
- Prepare the ingredients: The onion should be sautéed. Squeeze, cut, and thaw the spinach. Cook and cut up the bacon. Cut the roasted bell pepper into dice.
- Add the spices, salt, and pepper after beating the eggs.
- Mix together all the ingredients in a big bowl.
- Fill the baking dish with oil and pour in the mixture. When a toothpick inserted in the center comes out clean, bake for 30 to 40 minutes.

BREADCRUMB-FREE CRAB CAKES

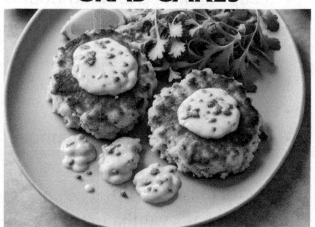

Servings: 6
Ingredients

- ½ head of cauliflower, rinsed, steamed, and water extracted (1 cup when finished)
- 5 free-range eggs
- 3 tablespoons Garlic Avocado Aioli (Store-bought is fine)
- ¼ cup finely chopped curly parsley
- ½ teaspoon sea salt

- ¼ teaspoon ground pepper
- ½ teaspoon cayenne pepper
- ½ teaspoon paprika
- 1 teaspoon fresh dill
- 6 tablespoons coconut flour
- 1 pound responsibly sourced crabmeat, cooked
- 2 tablespoons avocado oil or coconut oil (for searing)
- Lemon juice to taste

Directions:

- Use a strong blender or food processor to rice the cauliflower. Ten minutes of steaming. Use cheesecloth, a kitchen towel, or a nut milk bag to press out any remaining liquid. Leave it to cool.
- In a small dish, whisk together the eggs, Garlic Avocado Aioli, and seasonings.
- In a medium-sized bowl, gently fold in the cooled cauliflower, egg mixture, and coconut flour until well combined. (The cauliflower must be cold in order to prevent cooking the eggs.) The crab cakes' completed exterior is lovely and crispy thanks to the cauliflower and coconut flour.
- Take care not to tear up the flesh too much as you gently fold in the crabmeat. (It is preferable if the finished crab cakes contain sizable pieces of meat.)
- After 15 minutes of refrigeration, cool the mixture and preheat the oven to 350°F.
- Patties should be about 1 inch thick and 3 inches wide.
- Transfer oil into a cast-iron pan (which is preferable) and place it over medium-high heat.
- Once the pan and oil are heated, carefully add the crab cakes, taking care not to pack the pan too full as this would result in steaming rather than searing.
- After about three minutes of cooking, turn the crab cakes over and continue cooking for an additional three minutes.
- After transferring the pan-fried crab cakes to a baking sheet, bake them for a full 12 to 15 minutes. To taste, drizzle the patties with lemon juice.

CHICKEN NUGGETS

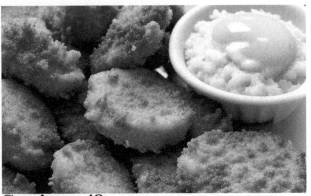

Servings: 48

Ingredients

- 8 boneless, skinless free-range hormone-free chicken breasts
- 3 cups quinoa flour
- 2 teaspoons garlic powder
- 2 teaspoons sea salt
- 2 teaspoons ground black pepper
- 4 eggs, beaten
- 1 cup coconut oil

Directions:

- Cut the chicken into bits the size of nuggets—roughly six pieces for each breast of chicken.
- In shallow dish, firmly mix flour, garlic powder, salt, and pepper.
- After dipping each chicken piece separately into the beaten eggs, lightly dust both sides with the flour mixture.
- Transfer the chicken to a plate, shaking off any excess flour, and repeat until all of the chicken is covered.
- Use a lot of coconut oil to generously coat a large, nonreactive skillet or saucepan (cast iron is my fave). Use just enough to keep the chicken nuggets from becoming dry in parts, but not too much that they become mushy.
- The nuggets should be sautéed for 4 minutes on each side or until golden brown. Between batches, you might need to take a moment to quickly clear the pan of any remaining tiny parts. If you don't, those bits burn easily and create unfavorable conditions for the fresh nuggets.
- When the core of your nuggets is no longer pink and they are a golden brown, you will know they are done. Each batch will take roughly 12 minutes.

PURPLE GOLD KRAUT

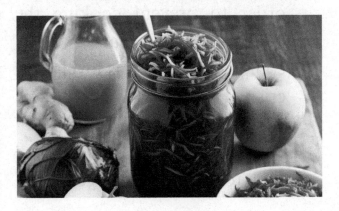

Servings: 14 Cups

Ingredients

- 2 heads of organic red cabbage, shredded
- ⅓ cup fresh organic turmeric, finely grated
- ⅓ cup fresh organic ginger, finely grated
- 2 tablespoons sea salt
- 2 tablespoons apple cider vinegar
- Additional brine
- 4 cups purified water
- 4 teaspoons sea salt
- 4 teaspoons apple cider vinegar

Directions:

- Remove four to five sizable leaves from one cabbage head and reserve. Cut up the leftover cabbage.
- In a large bowl, combine the shredded cabbage, ginger, turmeric, salt, and vinegar. (Use a stainless steel bowl so as not to have glaring yellow discoloration from the turmeric.)
- Put on gloves to prevent staining your hands and use your hands to massage the cabbage mixture until it begins to break down and soften, which should take five to ten minutes.
- To allow the combination to continue macerating and releasing more juices, let it sit for a duration of 20 to 30 minutes.
- For an additional five to ten minutes, massage the mixture.
- Using a big, long-handled spoon, fill two 36-ounce mason jars with the cabbage mixture. Tightly pack the mixture into the container until the very bottom.
- Brine, or the natural juices produced during the maceration process, is what you want to immerse the combination in. A gap of roughly 1½ inches should be left from the jar's top.
- Usually, more brine will need to be made. To achieve this, mix water, apple cider vinegar, and sea salt. Add more brine until the cabbage mixture is completely covered.
- To force the cabbage beneath the brine, roll up the reserved cabbage leaves and put them inside the jar.

- Loosely screw on the jar lid to let gas to escape throughout the fermentation process. Place in a cool, shaded spot on the counter for a period of 5 to 14 days.
- The sauerkraut will start to cloud and bubble during fermentation. Replace with fresh cabbage leaves to keep the cabbage submerged if scum or mold develops on the top of the leaves or throughout.
- Each day, taste the sauerkraut. Once you are satisfied with the taste, take off the rolled-up cabbage leaves and refrigerate the sauerkraut to slow down the fermenting process.

Tip:
- When preparing this meal, use gloves and easily-stainsorable clothing because the turmeric juice can discolor your hands and possibly leave lasting stains on them.
- Fruit that speeds up the fermenting process, like pineapple, may help you get the flavor you want faster. The sauerkraut is crisp and very fresh after 5 to 6 days. The flavor becomes slightly tarter and the texture becomes softer after about ten days. This sauerkraut goes really well with a dish for breakfast.

YELLOW CAULIFLOWER TORTILLAS

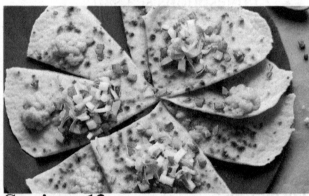

Servings: 12
Ingredients
- 2 heads of cauliflower, steamed (yields approximately 8 cups chopped cauliflower)
- 1 cup chopped green onions (approximately 2 bunches)
- 5 large free-range eggs, beaten
- ½ teaspoon sea salt
- ½ teaspoon finely ground black pepper
- ½ teaspoon ground turmeric
- ¾ teaspoon xanthan gum

Directions:
- Set oven temperature to 350°F.
- The cauliflower heads should be steamed for 4 to 5 minutes, or until soft.

- In a food processor or strong blender, blend the cauliflower and green onions until smooth (the onions will give them a small green tint, but that will change to yellow when you add the turmeric). About 32 fluid ounces should be produced from this mixture.
- To remove any extra liquid, strain the mixture using cheesecloth or a nut milk bag.
- In a medium bowl, stir together the cauliflower mixture, eggs, xanthan gum, salt, and pepper.
- For each tortilla, transfer ¼ cup of batter onto a baking sheet that has been prepared with silicone baking liners or parchment paper.
- Bake just one side for twenty-five minutes.
- Remove off the baking sheet and let cool.

FRESH MINT AND PEA SPREAD

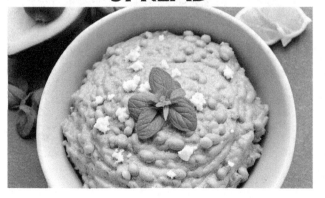

Servings: 24
Ingredients
- 3 cups fresh English peas
- ½ cup almonds, ground to consistency of flour
- Zest of 1 lemon
- 2 cups fresh mint, well packed
- 3 tablespoons lemon juice
- 1 shishito pepper
- 2 ounces goat cheese
- ½ cup avocado oil

Directions:
- In a strong blender, combine all the ingredients and process on medium speed until the spread reaches the appropriate consistency.
- Keep in a glass container and refrigerate. The spread keeps for five to seven days in the refrigerator.

MEYER LEMON–GINGER SALMON

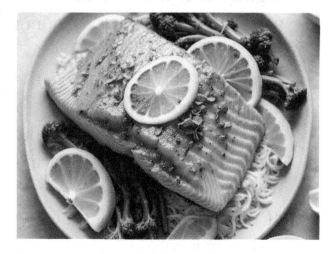

Servings: 12

Ingredients

- 1 to 2 tablespoons sesame oil
- 1 large wild salmon fillet (2½ to 3 pounds)
- 2 tablespoons low-sodium organic miso
- 1 tablespoon coconut aminos
- 4 tablespoons grated fresh ginger
- ½ teaspoon grated fresh turmeric
- 2 teaspoons minced garlic
- 2 teaspoons raw local honey
- Juice from 2 large Meyer lemons
- Zest from 3 large Meyer lemons

Directions:

- Set oven temperature to 350°F.
- Before you place the salmon in it, skin-side down, prepare a big baking dish (15 inches is the ideal size).
- Lightly coat the bottom of the pan with sesame oil. (By doing this, the skin won't stick.)
- In a small bowl, combine the other ingredients and stir to make a thick sauce. Spoon the fish with the sauce. (During baking, the thick, zesty portion of the sauce will remain on top and form a crust; the fluids, on the other hand, will slide to the bottom of the pan and flavor and moisten the remaining fish.)
- Bake the salmon for about 45 minutes, or until the thickest portion of the fillet is cooked through and the top begins to brown.

Tip:

- You can trim off the salmon's little tail end and place it in the empty space in the baking dish if your fillet is too long for it; it doesn't have to cook in one piece.
- Keep an eye on the salmon's thinner sections to make sure they don't overcook and get dry; if necessary, remove them early.

BRAISED BEEF COLLAGEN BOOST

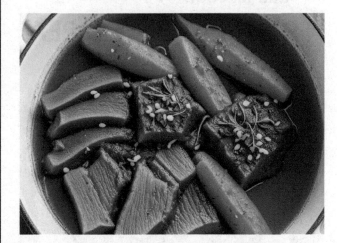

Servings: 12

Ingredients

- 4 to 4½ cups beef bone broth
- 8 pounds organic grass-fed beef
- 1 tablespoon sea salt for searing
- 1 tablespoon ground black pepper for searing
- 1 onion, peeled and cut into 8 wedges
- 12 ounces tomato paste (buy only brands that come in glass containers)
- 2 cups carrots (3 to 4 large carrots, cut into 2-inch chunks)
- 4 celery stalks, cut into 2-inch-long chunks
- 1 tablespoon ground herbes de Provence
- 4 to 5 whole garlic cloves

Directions:

- This recipe is meant to be used with a 6-plus-quart slow cooker.
- Bring the bone broth in your slow cooker to a simmer. I occasionally boil the bone broth before using it.
- Season all surfaces with salt and pepper before searing your beef.
- Turn up the heat to medium-high in a big frying or sauté pan and sear the meat until it turns a light golden brown on both sides.
- This is a crucial phase because it involves two processes that will combine to create a tasty final dish: flavor development and moisture retention. The flavor of all the crispy bits will permeate your braising liquid.
- Add the meat to the slow cooker along with all the other ingredients. Let it braise for four to eight hours. (I cook it for the whole eight hours to ensure that the meat is really soft and ready to eat when my workday is over.)

Tips:

- In the morning, use a 6 ½-quart slow cooker. The longer the flavors combine, the better braised meats taste, and it's like getting a free dinner without having to spend any time preparing it.
- This recipe makes enough to feed a small army because of this: eat some, freeze some, and share some!
- Transfer 1½ cups of the sauce to a pot before serving if you would like to have some sauce to go with your braised beef.

- Using a little whisk, combine 1 to 2 teaspoons of arrowroot powder with a small amount of warm liquid in a small glass. Next, add this mixture to the pot with the sauce you reserved. This method of premixing reduces clumping.

SALMON IN PARCHMENT PAPER

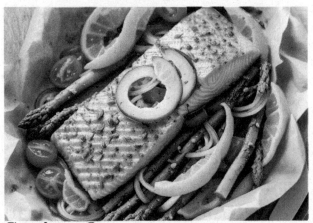

Servings: 8
Ingredients
- 16 ounces asparagus
- 2 yellow bell peppers, thinly sliced
- 1 red onion, thinly sliced
- 4 large tomatoes, diced
- 4 tablespoons capers, drained
- 8 salmon fillets
- 2 lemons, juiced
- ¼ cup avocado oil
- 3 lemons, sliced
- 1 teaspoon sea salt
- 1 teaspoon ground pepper
- ½ teaspoon cayenne pepper
- ½ cup basil, thinly sliced

Directions:
- Set oven temperature to 400°F.
- Cut eight 17-inch squares out of the parchment paper.
- Among the eight parchment squares, distribute the asparagus, bell peppers, onions, tomatoes, and capers equally.
- Top each with 1 salmon fillet. Over each piece of salmon, drizzle a little avocado oil and lemon juice.
- Add one or two lemon slices, salt, pepper, and a sprinkling of cayenne on top. Place the sides of the parchment paper over the salmon and fold them twice to create airtight pockets by sealing them.
- The pockets should be put on a baking pan.
- Bake the salmon for 15 to 20 minutes; when you stick your thermometer through the paper and into the fish, it should read 140°F to 145°F. Cut open each packet by placing it on a different plate. Serve the fish right away after sprinkling some basil on top.

Tips:

- The fish retains its moisture content and flavor thanks to the parchment paper!
- This dish is a hit with dinner guests as well because it presents well when served in the parchment paper

GREEN BEANS WITH CARAMELIZED SHALLOTS

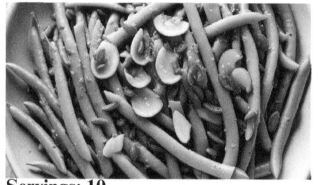

Servings: 10

Ingredients

- 15 shallots
- 1 to 2 tablespoons avocado oil
- 2 pounds green beans
- 1 cup sliced almonds
- 2 tablespoons grass-fed butter
- 1 teaspoon salt
- ½ teaspoon pepper

Directions:

- Peel and thinly slice the shallots to prepare them. In a medium-sized frying pan, place the shallots and 1 tablespoon of the avocado oil.

- Sauté the shallots until they are caramelized and golden brown, which could take up to 30 minutes.
- If needed, add more oil. Stir from time to time, but not too frequently, as the shallots require time to cook and frequent stirring will prevent the caramelization from occurring.
- However, be sure to keep a close check on them to prevent burning. When the shallots are caramelized, set them aside in a bowl.
- Get the beans ready for a blanch. Pour enough water into an 8-quart stockpot to cover the beans. Trim the ends of the beans and set them aside while the water heats.
- After blanching the beans, fill a large bowl with ice and cold water to create an ice bath. To halt the cooking process, immediately move the beans from the stockpot to the ice bath after they have been boiling for about three minutes.
- After the beans have cooled, take them out of the ice bath, reserve, and drain.

- Almond slices should be gently toasted in a skillet over medium heat. To liberate the oils and provide an extra-nutty flavor, the nuts should be lightly browned.
- In a large sauté or frying pan, melt the butter over medium-high heat five minutes before serving. To the butter in the pan, add the green beans, salt, and pepper.
- Add the sliced almonds and caramelized shallots to the heated beans. Evenly combine and proceed to serve.

CARDAMOM CARROT FRIES

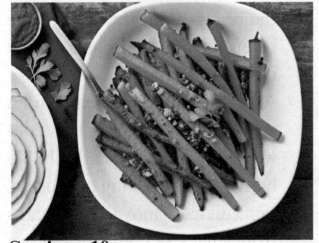

Servings: 10

Ingredients

- 8 cups carrot sticks (start with 6 pounds large organic carrots)
- 2 tablespoons avocado oil
- 3 teaspoons ground herbes de Provence
- 1½ teaspoons chili powder
- 2 tablespoons cardamom (adjust to taste)
- ¼ teaspoon cayenne pepper
- 1½ teaspoons salt
- ¼ teaspoon pepper

Directions:

- Set oven temperature to 375°F.
- After pealing the carrots, chop them into uniform lengths to begin making "fries." Next, remove the carrots' rounded corners by "square off" the carrots.
- After the carrots are arranged in square columns, cut them into the required fry thickness. Cut these slices into fries.
- In a big bowl, combine the avocado oil and the carrot fries, tossing to coat evenly. Toss to evenly mix the remaining ingredients.
- Use parchment paper or nonstick baking liners to line two large baking sheets.
- Make sure the fries are arranged so they don't touch. The best results will come from giving each fry enough room to allow for even browning.
- Bake for 30 to 45 minutes,

- monitoring to make sure they are cooking evenly about every 10 minutes.

SPICY ZUCCHINI APPLE MUFFINS

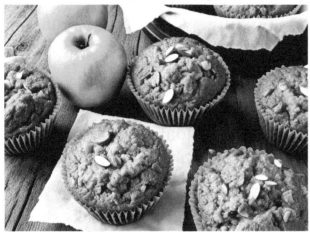

Servings: 24

Ingredients

- 2 cups grated zucchini
- 2 cups grated green apple
- 6 Medjool dates
- 1 cup nut butter
- 4 eggs
- ¼ cup coconut oil, melted
- 3 teaspoons vanilla extract
- 1 cup almond flour
- 1 teaspoon baking powder
- ½ teaspoon baking soda
- 4 teaspoons ground cinnamon
- 1 teaspoon ground ginger
- 1 teaspoon freshly ground nutmeg
- ¾ teaspoon allspice
- ¾ teaspoon ground cloves
- ½ teaspoon salt

Directions:

- Set oven temperature to 350°F.
- Peel and grate the apple and zucchini. Take out as much juice from the zucchini as you can.
- Using a mortar and pestle, smash the dates and remove the pits, or pulse them in a food processor until they become a paste.
- In a large bowl, blend the nut butter, eggs, and smashed dates. Blend in the apple, zucchini, coconut oil, and vanilla until well combined.
- Transfer the remaining ingredients to another bowl and stir to combine.
- Stir the dry mixture into the wet mixture just until combined.
- Give a silicone muffin pan or silicone muffin cups a light oiling. Just line the muffin tin with paper liners if silicone is not available. Pour a quarter of a cup of batter into each cup.
- A toothpick inserted into the center of the muffins should come out clean after 15 to 20 minutes of baking.

ALMOND COCONUT BREAD

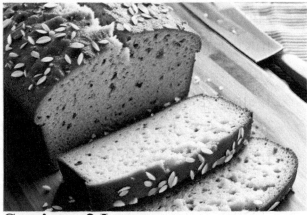

Servings: 2 Loaves

Ingredients

- 2 cups almond flour
- 1½ cups coconut flour
- ⅔ cup hemp seeds
- ½ cup ground flaxseed
- ½ cup whole psyllium husks
- 2 tablespoons baking powder
- 2 teaspoons ground anise seed (optional, or spice of choice)
- 2 teaspoons salt
- 12 eggs, room temperature
- 1 cup raw cheddar cheese, grated
- ⅔ cup coconut oil, melted
- 1½ cups raw-milk kefir

Directions:

- Set oven temperature to 350°F.
- In a large basin, combine all the dry ingredients. To uniformly mix the seeds, give it a good stir.
- In a large, separate bowl, beat the eggs. Add the other wet ingredients and beat until a homogeneous mixture forms.
- Gradually stir the dry ingredients into the wet mixture. (If the coconut oil clumps a little, this will disappear when baking.)
- Stir well. Transfer the mixture into two loaf pans coated with oil and backed with parchment paper.
- An inserted toothpick should come out clean after 45 to 50 minutes of baking.
- After taking the loaves out of the oven, take them out of the pans and immediately cool them on a cooling rack to allow the crust to dry; if the bread cools in the pan, it will get mushy.
- Before slicing, allow the loaves to cool completely. You can either slice and toast it immediately away, or slice and freeze it.

KALE CHIPS

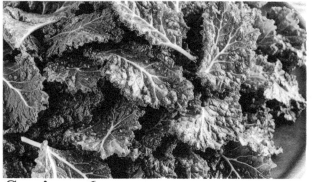

Servings: 6

Ingredients

- ½ pound curly kale leaves
- 2 tablespoons avocado oil
- Sea salt, to taste
- Add other spices such as cayenne or cinnamon to spice it up if desired

Directions:

- Turn the oven on to 425°F.
- Take off the kale's stiff stems. After washing and drying, cut the leaves into little pieces and transfer them to a large basin.
- After drizzling the kale with avocado oil, massage the oil into the leaves.
- Arrange the kale leaves uniformly on a baking sheet that has been lined, then bake.
- Using a spatula, separate any kale leaves that are sticking together at the 5-minute mark.
- Bake the kale for an additional 12 minutes or so, or until the leaves are crisp.
- Take out of the oven and lightly dust with salt.

FLAXSEED-CRUSTED SALMON WITH A ROASTED SQUASH AND BROCCOLI SALAD

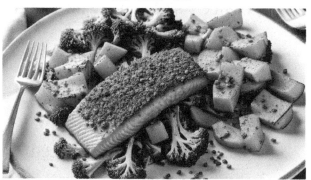

Servings: 4

Ingredients

Salad

- 1 small butternut squash, seeds removed, peeled and cubed
- 4 cups broccoli florets
- ⅓ cup olive oil, divided
- Sea salt, Freshly ground pepper
- 2 large lemons, juiced and zested
- 2 tablespoons champagne or white wine vinegar
- 2 teaspoons Dijon mustard
- 1 bunch Tuscan kale, washed, stems removed, and chopped

- One 14.5-ounce can cannellini or navy beans, drained and rinsed
- 2 medium Gala apples, cored and sliced thin
- 1 small shallot, halved and sliced thin
- ¼ cup roasted pumpkin seeds

Salmon

- 8-ounce skin-on wild-caught salmon fillet, patted dry
- 1 teaspoon olive oil
- 1 teaspoon Dijon mustard
- 1 garlic clove, grated
- 2 teaspoons ground flaxseed
- 2 thyme sprigs, leaves removed and minced
- ½ teaspoon sea salt
- ¼ teaspoon freshly ground black pepper

Directions:

- Set oven temperature to 400°F.
- After lining a large rimmed baking sheet with parchment paper, arrange the broccoli and squash on top.
- Over the vegetables, drizzle two to three tablespoons of olive oil. Add salt and pepper for seasoning, then transfer to the oven.
- Roast the vegetables for 20 to 25 minutes, or until they are soft to the fork. Take out of the oven and place somewhere to cool.
- With the skin side facing down, lay the salmon on a small, rimmed baking sheet that has been lined with parchment paper.
- In a small bowl, mix together the garlic, mustard, and teaspoon of olive oil.
- Mix thoroughly, then equally apply to the salmon fillet's top and sides.
- In a small bowl, combine the flaxseed, thyme, salt, and pepper.
- Press the mixture gently into the fish's mustard-glazed flesh.
- Fish should flake easily with a fork and be cooked through after about ten minutes of baking in the oven.
- As the salmon cooks, put the salad together.
- In a separate dish, mix together the lemon zest and juice, vinegar, mustard, and leftover olive oil. After whisking, taste and add salt and pepper as needed.
- In a big bowl, mix together the kale, beans, apple, shallot, and

- pumpkin seeds.
- Add the roasted vegetables that have slightly cooled. Pour the zesty vinaigrette on top and mix thoroughly.
- Accompany the salmon with a generous portion of salad.

PUMPKIN CHICKPEA CURRY STEW

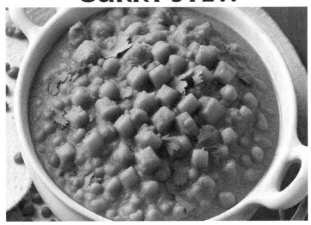

Servings: 4

Ingredients

- 2 tablespoons olive oil
- 1 large onion, diced
- 8 garlic cloves, minced
- 1 medium Fresno or jalapeño pepper, seeded and finely chopped
- 2 tablespoons freshly grated ginger
- One 14.5-ounce can pumpkin puree
- 2 teaspoons ground turmeric
- 1½ teaspoons sea salt
- 1 teaspoon cumin
- 1 teaspoon coriander
- 1 teaspoon freshly ground black pepper
- One 28-ounce can crushed tomatoes
- 2 to 3 cups vegetable broth
- 10 ounces fingerling potatoes, quartered
- One 14.5-ounce can chickpeas, drained and rinsed
- 2 cups frozen peas One
- 14.5-ounce can full-fat coconut milk
- 4 cups spinach
- 1½ cups quinoa, prepared according to the package directions
- ¼ cup plain coconut milk yogurt 1 lime, cut into wedges

Directions:

- In a big pot, warm the olive oil over medium heat.
- After adding the onion, sauté it for two to three minutes, or until it starts to become translucent.
- Stir together the ginger, garlic, and pepper after adding them. Cook, stirring gently, for an additional two minutes.
- Next, mix in the turmeric, salt, pepper, coriander, cumin, and pureed pumpkin.

- Simmer the mixture for 3 to 5 minutes, or until it starts to smell aromatic. Stir in the two cups of broth and the tomatoes.
- Add the potatoes and chickpeas after thoroughly stirring to ensure that all the particles from the bottom of the saucepan are included.
- Repeatedly stir. If the potatoes and beans aren't completely covered by the liquid, gradually add more broth until they are.
- After bringing to a slow boil, turn down the heat. Fork-tender potatoes should be achieved by simmering the saucepan covered for 25 to 30 minutes.
- After the potatoes get soft, take off the lid and mix in the spinach, peas, and coconut milk.
- Let the spinach wilt by gently stirring it over the heat. If necessary, add extra salt and pepper after tasting the stew.
- Spoon some cooked quinoa on top of the stew. Add some yogurt and a wedge of lime for squeezing on the side as garnish.

SESAME GINGER–ROASTED CHICKEN AND SWEET POTATO WITH A FENNEL AND PICKLED BEET SALAD

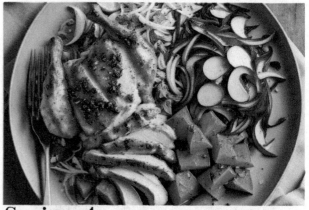

Servings: 4

Ingredients

Chicken and sweet potato

- 1 tablespoon toasted sesame oil
- 2 tablespoons avocado oil
- ¼ cup coconut aminos
- 2 tablespoons freshly grated ginger
- 1 teaspoon fish sauce (optional)
- 4 garlic cloves, minced
- 1½ teaspoons sea salt
- 1 teaspoon freshly ground black pepper
- One 8-ounce chicken breast, cubed
- 1 large sweet potato (or 2

medium), peeled and cubed

- 1 large onion, cut into
- 1½-inch-thick wedges
- 1 tablespoon sesame seeds
- Salad
- ¼ cup olive oil
- 3 tablespoons apple cider vinegar
- 1 small shallot, minced
- Sea salt
- Freshly ground black pepper
- 3 cups arugula
- 2 cups baby kale
- 3 small fennel bulbs, trimmed and sliced thin
- 2 cups pickled beet slices, cut into bite-size pieces
- 2 cups broccoli slaw mix
- 2 small Granny Smith apples, cored and sliced thin
- 2 tablespoons slivered almonds

Directions:

- Set oven temperature to 400°F.
- Line a baking sheet's rim with parchment paper.
- The first 8 ingredients for the chicken should be combined and thoroughly whisked together in a large basin.
- Toss to ensure even coating of the cubed chicken, sweet potato, and onion in the bowl

containing the sesame-ginger combination.

- Evenly distribute the chicken and veggies on the sheet pan.
- Any remaining marinade should be kept in the bowl.
- Roast the pan for fifteen minutes after placing it in the oven. Take the pan out of the oven for a little while, then evenly sprinkle the sesame seeds over the chicken and veggies and spray them with the remaining marinade.
- Cook the potatoes for a further 20 to 25 minutes, or until fork tender, after returning the pan to the oven.
- Make the salad while you wait for the chicken and veggies to be done.
- In a small bowl, whisk together the olive oil, vinegar, and shallot. To taste, add salt and pepper for seasoning.
- Combine the rest of the ingredients in a large serving bowl.
- Add the vinaigrette to the salad right before serving. Present the salad with the sweet potatoes and roasted chicken

CHIPOTLE BLACK BEAN–STUFFED SWEET POTATOES WITH CILANTRO-LIME CABBAGE SLAW

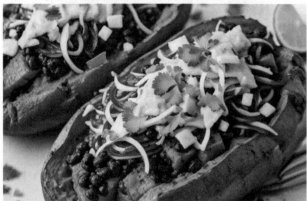

Servings: 4

Ingredients

Sweet potatoes

- 4 large sweet potatoes, washed and holes poked with fork or knife
- 2 tablespoons olive oil
- 1 red onion, diced
- 4 ounces tempeh, crumbled
- 6 garlic cloves, minced
- 1 chipotle pepper in adobo sauce, finely chopped
- One 14.5-ounce can diced tomatoes
- One 14.5-ounce can black beans, drained and rinsed
- 1 cup quinoa, rinsed
- 2 teaspoons sea salt
- 1 teaspoon freshly ground black pepper
- 1 teaspoon cumin
- 1 teaspoon chili powder
- ½ teaspoon paprika
- ¼ teaspoon cayenne pepper

Slaw

- 2 large limes, juiced
- 4 tablespoons plain coconut milk yogurt
- 1 tablespoon avocado oil
- 2 cups shredded cabbage (green or red)
- ½ white onion, sliced thin
- 1 small bunch cilantro, trimmed and chopped
- 1 avocado, pitted and cubed
- Sea salt
- Freshly ground black pepper
- 2 tablespoons ground flaxseeds
- 2 tablespoons roasted pumpkin seeds

Directions:

- Turn the oven on to 425°F.
- Place the prepped sweet potatoes on top of a baking sheet that has been lined with foil or parchment paper.
- Bake for approximately fifty minutes, or until the thickest part of the potatoes is fork-tender.
- Make the slaw after putting the sweet potatoes in the oven.

- In a small bowl, mix together the yogurt, oil, and lime juice. Once combined, whisk and set aside.
- In a medium or large bowl, mix together the avocado, cabbage, onion, and cilantro. Overtop, drizzle the lime-coconut mixture and toss to blend.
- Toss again after adding salt and pepper to taste. While you continue cooking, cover the bowl with plastic wrap and refrigerate to allow the flavors to mingle.
- Two tablespoons of olive oil are heated over medium-high heat in a big skillet.
- Add the onion and sauté for two to three minutes, or until it begins to become translucent.
- Cook the crumbled tempeh until it starts to get browned.
- After the tempeh begins to brown, add the minced garlic and sauté for an additional minute.
- Next, add the remaining ingredients, ranging from cayenne pepper to chipotle pepper.
- To ensure that the quinoa has enough moisture to cook, add 1½ cups of water.
- After the mixture starts to gently boil, reduce the heat to medium-low and whisk occasionally.
- The quinoa should start to open and curl after 15 to 20 minutes of cooking under cover, or when the sweet potatoes are ready to be taken out of the oven.
- Lower the heat to the lowest setting to maintain a gently simmer if the quinoa-bean mixture starts to boil before the potatoes are done.
- As necessary, taste and adjust the salt and pepper.
- When the sweet potatoes are cooked, make a slit in the middle to let out the steam, being cautious not to cut through the bottom layer of skin. To fluff up the centers, gently pinch the sides.
- Take the slaw out of the fridge and add the pumpkin seeds and flaxseeds.
- Top the potatoes with a heaping helping of the cilantro-cabbage slaw and the quinoa-

- bean mixture.

SHRIMP SCAMPI AND A WARM BACON BALSAMIC SQUASH AND DANDELION SALAD

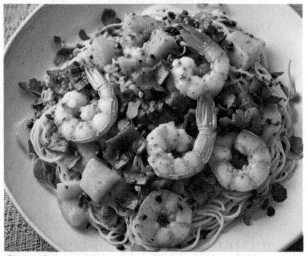

Servings: 4

Ingredients

Squash

- 1 large spaghetti squash, halved lengthwise and seeds removed
- Olive or avocado oil
- 1 large acorn squash, halved lengthwise and seeds removed
- Sea salt
- Freshly ground black pepper

Shrimp

- 2 tablespoons ghee
- 8 ounces wild-caught peeled and deveined shrimp

- 6 minced garlic cloves
- 1 teaspoon sea salt
- 1 teaspoon freshly ground black pepper
- ½ teaspoon red pepper flakes
- 2 lemons, juiced and zested
- 1 cup chicken broth
- 6 cups spinach
- 1 small bunch parsley, trimmed and chopped

Salad

- ¼ cup extra-virgin olive oil
- 3 tablespoons balsamic vinegar
- 1 tablespoon pure maple syrup
- Sea salt
- Freshly ground black pepper
- 2 thick-cut bacon slices, chopped
- 1 medium shallot, finely diced
- 4 cups dandelion greens or other bitter green (arugula, kale, radicchio)
- 1 cup bulgur or quinoa, cooked according to the package directions
- ¼ cup pomegranate seeds
- 2 tablespoons roasted sunflower or pumpkin seeds

Directions:

- Set oven temperature to 400°F.
- Put parchment paper on the bottom of a large baking sheet.
- After lightly sprinkling the flesh

of the spaghetti squash with oil and seasoning it with salt and pepper, set it flesh-side down on the baking sheet.

- Make a few holes in the top of each side using a fork or knife. Let it sit in the oven for 10 minutes.
- Complete the acorn squash's preparations while the spaghetti squash cooks.
- Peel the skin right away if you don't like its texture; else, let it alone. Slice each half into ½-inch pieces.
- Lightly oil each slice on all sides and sprinkle with a small amount of salt and pepper, much like you did with the spaghetti squash.
- Remove the spaghetti squash from the oven and place the acorn squash on the baking sheet when it has had its ten minutes of prep time.
- Place the sheet containing the two squashes back in the oven.
- Using a spatula, turn the acorn squash slices after another 10 to 15 minutes, and cook for a further 10 to 15 minutes, or until both squashes are soft.

- When finished, take the spaghetti squash out of the oven, turn it over so that additional steam may escape, and set it aside.
- Start preparing the shrimp (you may do this while you wait for the squash to complete or after it has rested).
- Heat the ghee in a big skillet over medium-high heat. Shrimp and garlic are added when the ghee has melted, and season with red pepper flakes, salt, and pepper.
- Sauté the shrimp, stirring now and then, until they are opaque and pink.
- Pour the broth in along with the lemon zest and juice. Lower the heat as soon as the liquids start to boil.
- Add the spinach and simmer until the liquids have reduced by half.
- Turn off the heat and carefully spoon the cooked spaghetti squash flesh into the mixture when the spinach has shrunk and wilted.
- The flesh of the squash should break apart resembling little noodles. Mix the ingredients

- thoroughly. As necessary, adjust the salt by tasting it.
- Proceed to complete the salad.
- Whisk the oil, vinegar, and maple syrup in a small basin. After adding salt and pepper to taste, reserve.
- Preheat a large skillet over medium-high heat.
- To ensure that all of the bacon cooks evenly, add the chopped bacon to the pan and stir from time to time.
- Add the shallots once the bacon is starting to crisp up around the edges and the majority of the fat has been rendered.
- Simmer the onion for an additional one to two minutes, or until it turns translucent.
- After turning off the heat, add the dandelion greens. When the greens are almost tender, pour the contents of the skillet into a big bowl.
- Stir in the roasted acorn squash, sunflower, pomegranate, and cooked bulgur. After tossing, drizzle with the balsamic vinaigrette.
- Top the scampi with finely

chopped parsley and present a substantial portion of the salad alongside.

GHEE-BASTED PORK CHOPS, SAUTÉED FENNEL, AND LEEKS WITH KALE AND ROASTED POTATOES

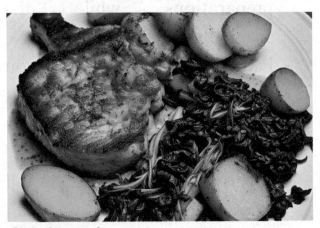

Servings: 4
Ingredients
Potatoes

- 1 pound fingerling (or baby) potatoes, washed and halved
- 2 medium turnips, washed and cubed (about the same size as the halved potatoes)
- 3 tablespoons ghee, melted
- 2 garlic cloves, grated
- 2 rosemary sprigs, leaves removed and minced
- 1½ teaspoons sea salt
- 1 teaspoon freshly ground black pepper

Fennel, leeks, and kale

- 3 tablespoons avocado oil
- 2 leeks, washed, roots and dark green tops trimmed, white and pale green parts sliced
- 1 lemon, sliced thin with seeds removed
- 3 large fennel bulbs, trimmed and sliced thin
- 1 teaspoon sea salt
- 1 teaspoon freshly ground black pepper
- ½ to 1 teaspoon red pepper flakes (½ teaspoon for milder spice, 1 teaspoon if you like more heat)
- 4 cups kale
- 1 14.5-ounce can cannellini or navy beans, drained and rinsed

Pork chop

- 4 thick-cut bone-in pork chops (8 to 10 ounces), patted dry
- Sea salt
- Freshly ground black pepper
- 2 fresh thyme sprigs, leaves removed and minced
- 1 tablespoon ghee, divided
- ¾ cup chicken broth

Directions:

- Set oven temperature to 400°F.
- Line a baking sheet's rim with parchment paper.
- In a sizable bowl, combine the potatoes, turnips, ghee, garlic, rosemary, salt, and pepper.
- Scatter the potato and turnip mixture evenly onto the baking sheet that has been prepared after everything has been well seasoned and moistened.
- After placing in the oven, cook for 25 to 30 minutes, or until the veggies are soft to the fork.
- Prepare the other vegetables while the potatoes are roasting.
- In a big skillet over medium-high heat, warm the avocado oil.
- Cook the leeks for 3 to 4 minutes, or until they begin to soften, after adding them.
- Cook for an additional few minutes after adding the lemon slices.
- Add the fennel and season with salt, pepper, and red pepper flakes after the leeks are transparent and the lemons are beginning to color on the edges.
- Kale and beans should be added when the fennel has begun to shrivel and soften.
- Simmer for a further three to four minutes, or until the beans are thoroughly heated and the

kale has begun to wilt. After tasting and adding additional salt if necessary, turn off the heat.

- Turn the heat up to medium-high in another skillet. Season the pork chops with salt, pepper, and minced thyme while the skillet is heating up.
- Pour half of the ghee into the skillet once it's heated. Once it has melted, include the pork chops.
- Without touching the pork, sear it for 5 minutes, then turn it over and continue to sear it for an additional 5 minutes.
- When the pork has seared on both sides, pour the leftover ghee into the skillet.
- Flip the pork chops with tongs and baste them with a spoon or heatproof basting brush, then glaze them with the pan's cooking juices and ghee.
- After about five minutes of flipping and basting, take the pork out of the skillet and let it rest for at least ten minutes.
- While using a whisk to scrape up all the fat (pork bits left on the bottom), pour the heated skillet's chicken stock into it to deglaze it.
- When the broth starts to boil, turn down the heat to medium-low and continue to gently simmer until at least half of the liquid has been reduced. If necessary, taste the reduction and add additional salt.
- After slicing the pork chops, top them with a generous portion of potatoes, sautéed veggies, and reduction sauce.

CHICKPEA PANCAKES WITH SAUTÉED BEANS AND GREENS WITH A LEMON TAHINI DRESSING

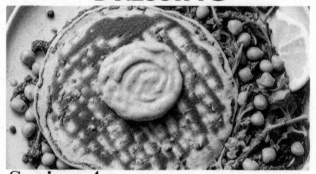

Servings: 4
Ingredients
Pancakes

- 4 cups chickpea flour (besan)
- ⅓ cup nutritional yeast
- 2 teaspoons sea salt
- 1 teaspoon freshly ground black pepper

- 1 teaspoon ground turmeric
- 1 teaspoon cumin
- ½ teaspoon coriander
- ½ teaspoon cayenne pepper
- 2½ cups water
- Avocado oil

Tahini dressing

- ⅓ cup tahini
- 1 large lemon, juiced and zested
- 1 garlic clove, grated
- Sea salt
- Freshly ground black pepper
- Beans and greens
- 3 tablespoons avocado oil, divided
- One 14.5-ounce can chickpeas, drained and rinsed
- ½ teaspoon sea salt
- ½ teaspoon freshly ground black pepper
- ½ teaspoon paprika
- ½ teaspoon cumin
- ¼ teaspoon crushed red pepper flakes
- 3 garlic cloves, grated
- 6 cups chopped kale

Toppings

- 1 cup pickled red onion
- 2 tablespoons toasted sesame seeds
- 2 tablespoons roasted pumpkin seeds
- 2 tablespoons whole flaxseeds

Directions:

- In a large bowl, mix together all of the pancake ingredients, excluding the oil.
- Mix the batter until it's smooth and free of lumps, then put it aside.
- In a small bowl, mix together all the ingredients for the tahini dressing.
- Once combined, whisk in a small amount of water at a time until the dressing achieves the desired consistency—it can be as thick or thin as desired. After adding salt and pepper to taste, reserve.
- In a sizable skillet, heat up 1½ tablespoons of avocado oil over medium-high heat. Stir in the red pepper, cumin, paprika, black pepper, and chickpeas. Move the beans from the pan and set them aside after cooking, stirring from time to time, until they start to get crispy and golden.
- Back in the skillet you used for the beans, add the remaining 1½ tablespoons of avocado oil and heat to medium-high.

- When the kale and garlic are added, season with a small pinch of salt and pepper.
- After the kale has wilted, turn off the heat and set it aside.
- Over medium heat, preheat a small or medium nonstick skillet.
- Add less than a tablespoon of oil, just enough to coat the pan's bottom.
- After giving the batter a short stir while it's resting, take out enough batter (about ½ cup) to almost completely cover the pan's bottom.
- Cook for 1 to 2 minutes, or until bubbles start to form, then carefully turn with a spatula and continue cooking for an additional 2 minutes, or until the pancake is cooked through and has a hint of golden color.
- After taking the pancake out of the griddle, set it aside. Continue doing this until all of the batter has been used.
- The pancakes should be served with the crispy chickpeas, kale, and tahini sauce on top. Sesame, pumpkin, and
- flaxseeds could be used as garnish.

WHITE BEAN AND KALE SOUP

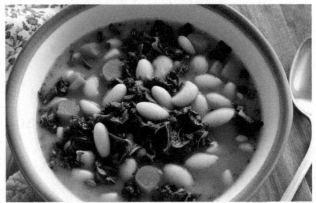

Servings: 4
Ingredients
- 2 tablespoons avocado oil
- 1 large onion, diced
- 4 garlic cloves, minced
- 2 celery stalks, chopped
- 2 medium carrots, peeled and chopped
- 2 fresh thyme sprigs, leaves removed and minced
- 3 fresh oregano sprigs, leaves removed and minced
- 1½ teaspoons sea salt
- 1 teaspoon freshly ground black pepper
- 1 teaspoon crushed red pepper flakes
- 5 cups vegetable broth
- Two 14.5-ounce cans cannellini or navy beans, drained and

rinsed

- 6 cups chopped kale
- 1 large lemon, cut into wedges

Directions:

- In a big pot, warm the oil over medium-high heat.
- After adding the onion, sauté it for about two minutes, or until it begins to turn transparent.
- Stir in the remaining 8 ingredients (red pepper flakes to garlic).
- After 3 more minutes of cooking with occasionally stirring, add the beans and broth.
- Mix well and heat on medium-high until the mixture starts to boil.
- Turn the heat down to low, taste, and adjust the salt if necessary. Cover and simmer the beans for 20 to 25 minutes to let the flavors seep in.
- In the final five minutes of simmering, add the kale to the soup and mix thoroughly to incorporate.
- Zest a lemon wedge and squeeze it over the soup before serving.

HERBY STEAKS WITH MASHED POTATOES AND ROASTED VEGGIE MEDLEY

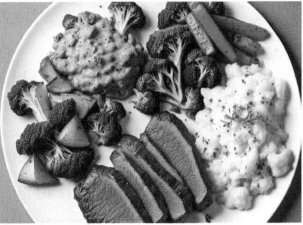

Servings: 4

Ingredients

Steak

- 10-ounce bone-in ribeye steak
- Sea salt
- 2 teaspoons avocado oil
- Freshly ground black pepper
- 1 tablespoon ghee
- 1 garlic clove, smashed
- 1 fresh thyme sprig
- 1 fresh oregano sprig

Roasted veggies

- ¼ cup avocado oil
- 4 cups broccoli florets
- 4 cups cauliflower florets
- 4 cups brussels sprouts, trimmed and halved
- 1½ teaspoons sea salt
- 1 teaspoon garlic powder

- 1 teaspoon freshly ground black pepper

Mashed potatoes

- 1 pound Yukon Gold potatoes, peeled and cubed
- Sea salt
- 3 tablespoons ghee
- ½ teaspoon ground white pepper (optional)
- Freshly ground black pepper

Directions:

- Set oven temperature to 400°F.
- Put parchment paper on the bottom of a large baking sheet.
- Take the steak out of the fridge and sprinkle salt on both sides.
- Let it cool to room temperature.
- In a large bowl, mix together all the ingredients for the roasted veggies.
- Mix until thoroughly seasoned and coated with oil.
- After transferring to the prepared baking sheet, bake the vegetables for 25 to 30 minutes, or until they are soft to the fork.
- Put the potatoes in a big pot and add water to cover them. Add salt to the water until it has a sea flavor.
- Remove from stovetop and drain after bringing to a boil over high heat and cooking until potatoes are fork tender.
- Place the strained potatoes back into the hot pot from earlier.
- Add the black pepper to taste, ghee, and white pepper, if using.
- Mash to the required level of consistency. After cooking in the seasoned water, the potatoes should be well-seasoned; however, taste them to make sure, and add additional salt if necessary.
- It's time to cook the steak when the potatoes are done and the roasted veggies are almost done.
- In a medium cast-iron skillet set over high heat, heat the oil and add a final dash of pepper to season the steak while it rests.
- Add the steak to the skillet after it's heated and the oil is shimmering. Sear the meat for 4 to 5 minutes, or until a good crust forms on the bottom, without moving it. After

flipping the steak, add the garlic, herbs, and ghee.

- Continue basting the steak with the garlic-herb ghee for the remaining 4 to 5 minutes, or until it achieves your desired doneness, using a spoon or heat-resistant basting brush.
- When the steak is done, take it from the heat source and let it rest for ten minutes.
- Then, slice it up and serve it with as much of the potatoes and roasted veggies as possible, along with any liquids that may have remained on the cutting board.

SEED-CRUSTED CAULIFLOWER STEAKS WITH ARUGULA CHIMICHURRI–DRESSED BEANS AND SWEET POTATO FRIES

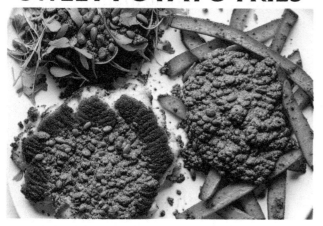

Servings: 4
Ingredients
Chimichurri and beans

- 2 garlic cloves, smashed
- 1 small shallot, peeled and roughly chopped
- ½ teaspoon crushed red pepper flakes
- 3 cups arugula
- 1 cup parsley
- ½ cup olive oil
- ⅓ cup red wine vinegar
- Sea salt
- Freshly ground black pepper
- One 14.5-ounce can chickpeas, drained (reserve bean liquid in cans) and rinsed

Fries

- 1 pound sweet potatoes, peeled and cut into relatively uniform ¼-inch-thick matchsticks
- 2 tablespoons avocado oil
- 2 teaspoons pure maple syrup
- 1 teaspoon cornstarch
- 1 teaspoon sea salt
- 1 teaspoon paprika
- ¼ teaspoon cayenne pepper
- Freshly ground black pepper

Cauliflower

- ⅓ cup nutritional yeast
- ¼ cup hemp seeds
- ¼ cup pumpkin seeds

- ¼ cup ground flaxseed
- 1 tablespoon chia seeds
- 2 teaspoons sea salt (use only 1 teaspoon if any of the seeds are pre-salted)
- 1 teaspoon freshly ground black pepper
- 1 teaspoon garlic powder
- 1 teaspoon onion powder
- Reserved canned chickpea liquid (aquafaba)
- 1 large head of cauliflower (or 2 medium), leaves removed, stem trimmed, and cut into 4 "steaks" about 1½ inches thick
- 2 tablespoons avocado oil

Directions:

- Turn the oven on to 425°F.
- Put parchment paper on both of the baking sheets' rims.
- Make the chimichurri beans first.
- In a food processor, combine first 5 ingredients; pulse until shallots and garlic are minced and greens are finely chopped. After adding the vinegar and olive oil, pulse a couple more times to combine the sauce.
- To taste, add salt and pepper for seasoning.
- In a large bowl, combine the chickpeas and chimichurri sauce; toss until the beans are well coated.
- Set aside to allow the flavors to mingle while preparing the remaining dishes.
- If you would rather the beans cold, you can store them in the refrigerator or leave them out at room temperature.

Get the fries ready now.

- In a large basin, toss the sweet potatoes with the oil and syrup until all the potatoes are well coated.
- In a small bowl, mix together the cornstarch, salt, paprika, cayenne, and black pepper.
- Cover the potatoes with a small amount of the cornstarch mixture. If there are any apparent white streaks in the fries, rub the cornstarch into them before tossing again to ensure fair distribution.
- Arrange the fries evenly on one of the baking sheets that has been prepped, then pop it into the oven.
- Bake the fries for ten to fifteen minutes, then turn them over with a spatula and continue

baking for an additional ten to fifteen minutes, or until the sides start to turn golden and crisp.

- Prepare the cauliflower while the fries are baking.
- In a clean food processor, combine the first nine ingredients and pulse until the seeds take on a thick, sandy texture.
- Spoon mixture into a small pie plate or baking sheet, ensuring it is evenly distributed.
- Make a little assembly line on your counter and put the reserved aquafaba, or chickpea juices, in a big shallow bowl or pie plate. The bowl containing aquafaba, the seed mixture, and the second baking sheet lined with parchment paper.
- It's time to coat the cauliflower. Carefully place a steak of cauliflower in the aquafaba.
- Make sure the liquid is properly soaked on all sides when you turn it over.
- After transferring the steak to the seed mixture, turn it over and gently press with your hands to coat all sides, then transfer it to the baking sheet.

- Continue doing this until all of the steaks are done.
- After giving the steaks a light oiling, put them in the oven.
- After cooking for 15 minutes, turn them over with a spatula and continue cooking for an additional 10 to 15 minutes, or until the cauliflower is soft and the crust is starting to become golden brown.
- During the final few minutes of the cauliflower's cooking process, if the fries have lost most of their heat, feel free to reheat them in the oven.
- Present the cauliflower steaks accompanied by a portion of sweet potato fries and a dollop of chimichurri chickpeas on top.

QUINOA TABOULI

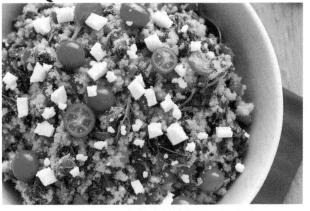

Servings: 6
Ingredients

- ½ cup quinoa
- 3 tablespoons lemon juice
- 2 tablespoons apple cider vinegar
- 1 tablespoon olive oil
- ½ teaspoon sea salt
- ½ teaspoon ground pepper
- 1 teaspoon ground herbes de Provence
- 1 cup spinach, chopped
- 1 cup cherry tomatoes, quartered
- 1 cup crumbled feta cheese
- 1 cup red bell pepper, diced

Directions:

- Follow the directions on the package to prepare the quinoa. In a big bowl, fluff and set aside to cool.
- You can prepare the salad dressing by combining lemon juice, apple cider vinegar, olive oil, sea salt, pepper, and herbs while the quinoa is cooking. Blend thoroughly and reserve.
- Assemble the remaining salad ingredients: Dice the bell peppers, chop the spinach, chop the tomatoes, and crumble the feta.
- After the quinoa cools, use a fork to fluff it once more. After adding and combining all the remaining ingredients, stir in the salad dressing very gently.
- Serve cold or store in the refrigerator for many hours or even overnight.

Tips:

- Rinsing the quinoa before cooking is an important step that keeps the grains apart and helps avoid clumping. This salad is a fantastic option if you're hosting a party and need to make a few dishes ahead of time because it tastes even better the next day.

BLACK AND ORANGE RICE

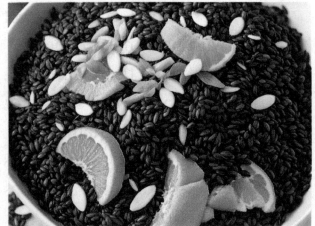

Servings: 7

Ingredients

- 2 cups black rice or wild rice blend
- 1¾ cups bone broth

- 4 tablespoons butter
- 1 cup scallions, thinly sliced (white and light green sections only)
- 1 cup sliced raw almonds
- Zest from 2 medium oranges
- 6 tablespoons freshly squeezed orange juice
- 1 teaspoon finely ground pepper
- Sea salt to taste

Directions:

- Follow the directions on the package to cook the wild rice.
- This is usually done on a simmer for 45 minutes after bringing the mixture to a rapid boil, using 2 cups of liquid for every cup of rice and butter.
- Make sure the rice is uniformly absorbing the broth by periodically checking on it.
- Prepare and measure the remaining ingredients (almonds, juice, cut scallions, and zest) and set them aside while the rice cooks.
- After the rice is cooked, combine the remaining ingredients and serve.

SWEET POTATO HASH BROWNS

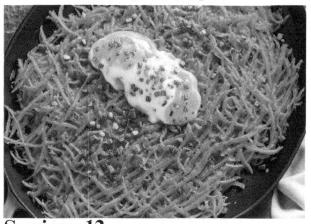

Servings: 12

Ingredients

- 3 cups shredded sweet potato
- 1 tablespoon salt (adjust to taste)
- 1 tablespoon pepper (adjust to taste)
- 1 teaspoon nutmeg
- 1 teaspoon allspice Grass-fed butter

Directions:

- Using a food processor or cheese grater, shred the sweet potato. (You can shred the sweet potato ahead of time to save time; it keeps well in the fridge for a few days.)
- In a larger bowl, mix together the salt, pepper, nutmeg, and allspice until well blended.
- In a frying pan over medium heat, melt the butter. Arrange a

few circular mounds of shredded sweet potato, each measuring ¼ cup, in the pan.

- Cook until done, 4 to 5 minutes on each side. The ideal texture is slightly crunchy on the outside and delicate on the inside.

ROASTED BUTTERNUT SQUASH SOUP

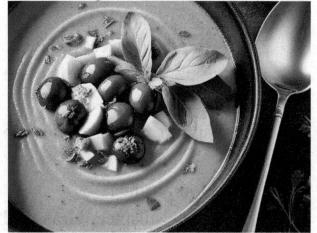

Servings: 6

Ingredients

- 4 cups butternut squash, cubed and roasted
- ½ onion, quartered and roasted
- ½ cup chestnuts, peeled and split in half
- 2 garlic cloves, smashed
- 3 tablespoons hazelnut oil
- 2½ cups bone broth
- 1 tablespoon raw apple cider vinegar
- ¼ teaspoon ground ginger
- ¼ teaspoon ground herbes de Provence
- 1/8 teaspoon cinnamon
- ¼ teaspoon salt
- 1/8 teaspoon pepper
- Dash cayenne pepper

Optional garnish

- 1 tablespoon crème fraîche added to the top of each serving
- 1 tablespoon fresh thyme, finely minced and sprinkled on each serving

Directions:

- Set oven temperature to 350°F.
- Butternut squash should be peeled, seeded, and cubed before being put in a glass baking dish or roasting pan.
- Add the onion half to the butternut squash after chopping it into four wedges.
- Add the crushed garlic cloves and the halves of chestnuts.
- Add hazelnut oil to the mixture and stir in the ginger, apple cider vinegar, cayenne, cinnamon, and herbes de Provence.
- Vegetables should be roasted for 45 minutes, or until they are soft and starting to turn brown.

- Measure out the other ingredients and set aside while the vegetables roast.
- When the veggies are ready, allow them to cool down a bit so handling them won't be as difficult.
- After the vegetables have cooled, put them in a strong blender or food processor. Blend in ½ cup of bone broth at a time. Add more bone broth until the soup reaches the right consistency.
- After transferring the soup to a big saucepan, heat it until it boils. Garnish with chosen toppings, if using.

Tip:
- To ensure that the veggies cook evenly and that the smaller pieces don't burn or overcook, use a baking dish or roasting pan that isn't too big. When processing hot food in a food processor or blender, use caution and gently open the lids to prevent explosions.

CACAO QUINOA CAKE

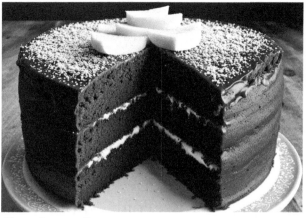

Servings: 8

Ingredients
- ⅔ cup quinoa
- ⅓ cup almond milk
- 1⅓ cups apple sauce
- ¾ cup coconut oil
- 2 teaspoons vanilla extract
- ¼ cup honey
- 2 eggs ⅓ cup coconut sugar
- 1 cup raw cacao powder
- 1½ teaspoons baking powder
- ½ teaspoon baking soda
- ½ teaspoon sea salt

Directions:
- To cook the quinoa, adhere to the package's instructions. (Normally, the directions ask for rinsing the quinoa grains, bringing them to a boil in 1⅓ cups of water, lowering the heat, simmering the grains for 10 minutes, letting them stand

- for 10 minutes, and letting them cool for 15 minutes.)
- Measure out all the ingredients and prepare an 8-inch square glass baking pan with coconut oil and greased parchment paper at the bottom while the quinoa cooks. Put aside.
- Set the oven to 350°F once the quinoa is cold enough to handle.
- Blend in three stages by pulsing in a food processor or strong blender. First, mix together the apple sauce, honey, coconut oil, vanilla extract, and almond milk.
- After that, mix in the eggs, coconut sugar, and cooked quinoa. Lastly, pulse in the salt, baking soda, baking powder, and cacao powder.
- After moving the cake to the baking dish, bake it for one hour and twenty-five minutes, or until a toothpick inserted in the center comes out clean.

Tip:
- You've never eaten a cake without gluten that is this moist! It seems like there is pudding in the cake

after everything is finished.
- Don't pulse the batter too much because the quinoa gives the finished baked cake a distinctive, somewhat crunchy texture and keeps it moist.

ROASTED TOMATO BISQUE

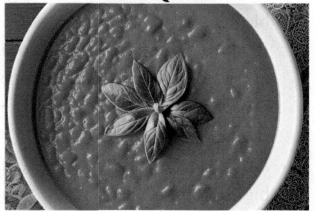

Servings: 4
Ingredients
- 4 tablespoons olive oil
- 8 medium Roma (plum) tomatoes
- 4 garlic cloves, minced
- 1 (15-ounce) can cannellini beans
- 2 cups chicken broth
- Salt and black pepper
- 1 cup heavy cream
- Fresh basil, julienned (optional)

Directions:
- Set oven temperature to 400°F. Apply a thin layer of olive oil

on a baking sheet to grease it.

- Cut the tomatoes in half, spread the garlic over them, and put them on the baking sheet.
- Roast the tomatoes for 20 to 25 minutes, or until they are tender.
- Place the beans in a blender along with the tomatoes and garlic.
- Process till everything is smooth.
- Fill a medium pot with the tomato-bean puree and place it over medium heat.
- After adding the broth and heating it through, taste and add salt and pepper as needed.
- After adding the cream, ladle the soup into separate bowls.
- If using, garnish with the basil and serve.

SHRIMP AND ASPARAGUS

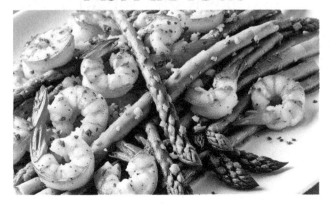

Servings: 4
Ingredients

- 2 tablespoons butter
- 2 tablespoons olive oil
- 1 pound shrimp, peeled and deveined
- 1 pound fresh asparagus, coarse ends trimmed and remainder sliced
- 1 tablespoon minced garlic
- Salt and black pepper
- Dash of smoked paprika (optional)
- ½ fresh lemon, zested and juiced
- ¼ cup (2 ounces) grated Parmesan cheese
- 2 tablespoons ground flaxseed

Directions:

- Melt the butter in a large skillet over medium heat, then drizzle with the olive oil.
- Add the shrimp and asparagus when the oil is shimmering, and sauté them for three to four minutes on low heat.
- After thoroughly stirring in the garlic, add the salt and pepper for seasoning.
- Pour in the paprika, if using, and then squeeze in the lemon juice and zest.

- Cook, stirring, over medium heat until the asparagus is soft and the shrimp is pink all the way through.
- In the meantime, mix the cheese and flaxseed together in a small bowl.
- When ready to serve, coat the shrimp and asparagus with the cheese-flaxseed mixture, swirl to combine, and then serve.

PUMPKIN AND CHICKEN CURRY WITH CAULIFLOWER RICE

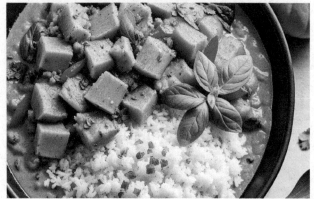

Servings: 4
Ingredients
- 2 tablespoons coconut oil
- 1 (4-ounce) skinless, boneless chicken breast or thigh, cubed
- ½ cup chopped red bell pepper
- ⅔ cup canned pumpkin puree
- Curry powder
- Other spices of choice
- 1 cup unsweetened coconut milk
- Fresh Thai basil, julienned
- 1 cup cauliflower rice, cooked according to package instructions

Directions:
- Melt and warm the coconut oil in a medium skillet over medium heat.
- After adding the chicken, simmer it for 3 to 4 minutes while stirring constantly, or until it is almost done.
- Incorporate the curry powder, pumpkin puree, red pepper, and your preferred spices. To thoroughly mix in the seasonings, stir the ingredients.
- Turn the heat up to medium-high, add the coconut milk, and boil. Simmer the food for ten minutes at a low temperature.
- Taste and adjust the spices accordingly. Spoon the curry into bowls and top with Thai basil. Accompany the cauliflower rice with it.

EGG AND VEGETABLE SALAD

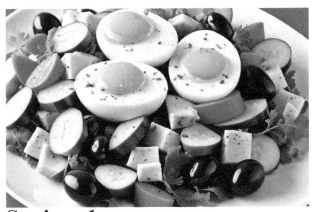

Servings: 1

Ingredients

- 2 hard-boiled large eggs, peeled and quartered
- 2 tablespoons olive oil mayonnaise or avocado oil mayonnaise
- 1 teaspoon spicy brown mustard
- 1 tablespoon apple cider vinegar
- ¼ cup sliced pitted olives
- 1 small cucumber, chopped
- 1 tablespoon diced red onion
- 1 celery stalk, diced
- 1 medium carrot, diced
- 2 large butter, bibb, or other lettuce leaves

Directions:

- Mash the eggs with the vinegar, mustard, and mayonnaise in a medium bowl. Mix thoroughly. Add the olives and stir.
- Combine the carrot, onion, celery, and cucumber in a

separate bowl.

- Place the lettuce leaves in a platter for serving. After adding the cucumber combination, spread the egg salad over it. Serve.

GRILLED CHICKEN SALAD

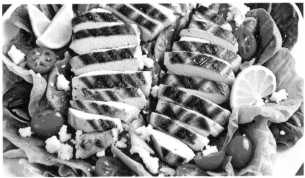

Servings: 4

Ingredients

- 4 cups water
- ¼ cup kosher salt
- 2 large boneless, skinless chicken breasts (about 1 pound), cut into 4 pieces
- 3 tablespoons olive oil, plus more for the grill
- 1 ½ teaspoons paprika
- 1 head romaine lettuce, chopped
- 1 lemon, juiced

Directions:

- In a large basin, combine the water and salt; mix to dissolve the salt. After adding the chicken to the bowl, chill it for half an hour.

- The chicken gains moisture from the brining.
- If you're using an outside grill, heat the grill on high for one side and medium for the other.
- As an alternative, heat a grill pan on the stovetop to medium-high.
- Dry off the chicken with a pat. Transfer the chicken breasts to a medium-sized bowl, drizzle with olive oil and paprika, and mix to coat.
- After lightly oiling the grill grates, put the chicken in the grill pan or on the hot side of the grill. Cook the chicken pieces without moving them until they begin to get grill marks.
- (Check by peering underneath.) Flip the pieces over and transfer them to the side of the grill that is colder (or lower the heat to medium beneath the grill pan). Grill the chicken until the thickest section registers 155°F on an instant-read thermometer.
- Cover the chicken with foil

after transferring it to a plate. Give it a ten-minute break.
- Place the romaine on a plate for serving. After setting the chicken over the romaine, drizzle with the lemon juice. Serve.

COTTAGE CHEESE OMELET

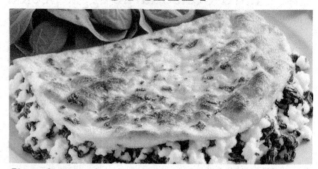

Servings: 1

Ingredients

- 2 large eggs
- 1 tablespoon milk
- Salt and black pepper
- 1 tablespoon olive oil
- ½ cup spinach
- 3 tablespoons full-fat cottage cheese

Directions:

- Mix the eggs, milk, and salt and pepper to taste in a medium-sized bowl, and whisk for 30 seconds.
- In a medium skillet set over medium heat, add the olive oil. Add the eggs when the oil is

shimmering and cook for one to two minutes, or until the eggs are mostly set.

- Spoon the cottage cheese and spinach onto half of the omelet after flipping it over.
- After cooking for a further one to two minutes, fold the omelet over the cottage cheese, and serve.

CONCLUSION

My heart is full of a mixture of feelings as this gastronomic journey draws to an end: appreciation, nostalgia, and a hint of bitter-sweetness. Yes, it has been quite the adventure. From the very first knife cut to the very last garnish flourish, we have laughed, faced difficulties, and experienced innumerable delectable moments together.

Looking through this cookbook reminds me of how food has the ability to nourish not only our bodies but also our souls. Every recipe has a backstory that revolves around love, relationships, and the everyday pleasures shared at the kitchen table.

A bowl of hot soup on a cold night or a rich dessert enjoyed with friends—food has the power to unite us and serve as a constant reminder of the important things in life.

Beyond the tastes and textures however, this cookbook is a celebration of strength and resiliency—the strength of women assisting one another through life's transformations and the resilience of women navigating the unknown seas of menopause. It serves as a reminder that preparing and enjoying a meal with loved ones can bring us comfort and joy, no matter what obstacles we encounter.

So let's take the spirit of this cookbook with us wherever we go as we say goodbye to these pages. One mouthwatering meal at a time, let's continue to celebrate the beauty of food, the strength of community, and the delight of living each moment to the fullest.

I hope your kitchens are full of

love, laughter, and the smells of delicious food shared with even greater people until we cross paths again, dear friends.

Bon Appétit

Made in the USA
Coppell, TX
13 November 2024

40132950R00050